"Send Us a Lady Physician"

WOMEN DOCTORS IN AMERICA, 1835-1920

*From various towns and cities we are
frequently receiving the inquiry,
"Can you not send us a reliable lady physician?"
—Dr. Ann Preston, 1864*

Edited by Ruth J. Abram

"Send Us a Lady Physician"

WOMEN DOCTORS IN AMERICA, 1835-1920

W.W. NORTON & COMPANY · New York · London

Sources frequently cited beneath photographs are identified by the following abbreviations: ASCWM, MCP = Archives and Special Collections on Women in Medicine, Medical College of Pennsylvania; NYAM = New York Academy of Medicine; and NLM = National Library of Medicine.

The text of this book is composed in Times Roman, with
display type set in Tiffany Demibold. Composition by PennSet, Inc.
Manufacturing by The Murray Printing Company.
Book design by Nancy Dale Muldoon.

First Edition

Library of Congress Cataloging in Publication Data
Main entry under title:
Send us a lady physician.
Includes index.
1. Women physicians—United States—History.
2. Medicine—United States—History. I. Abram, Ruth J.
[DNLM: 1. Physicians, Women—history—United States.
WZ 80.5.W5 S474]
R692.S46 1985   610′.92′2   85–13856

ISBN 0-393-02274-9

ISBN 0-393-30278-4 {PBK}

W. W. Norton & Company, Inc., 500 Fifth Avenue, New York, N.Y. 10110
W. W. Norton & Company Ltd., 37 Great Russell Street, London WC1B 3NU

1 2 3 4 5 6 7 8 9 0

Acknowledgments

*S*end Us a Lady Physician, was conceived over five years ago during a course I organized on women's history for leaders of national women's organizations. Taught by Gerda Lerner, Amy Swerdlow, and Alice Kessler Harris, this course confirmed me in my belief in the power of history as an organizing tool, as a vehicle for gaining social and political perspective, as a source of important role models, and as a goad for reform.

This project is a direct outgrowth of my involvement with the women's movement. It was within its embrace that I first perceived that all of us have a need and a right to the history of our groups. *Send Us a Lady Physician* is dedicated to the feminist movement, past, present, and future.

This book and the museum exhibit that it chronicles explore and interpret the history of women's entry into the American medical profession, the success they achieved by the century's end, and the difficulty they had maintaining a foothold in the profession in the early years of the twentieth century. By understanding this history, we may shed light on a critical question: How can any group outside the dominant culture first achieve and then sustain hard-won social, political, and economic gains? Because many variables change all the time, history does not really repeat itself. Therefore, we cannot expect to find exact parallels between the history told here and issues before us today. Still, there are insights to be gained, role models to be discovered, strategies to be considered, and the possibility of obtaining a perspective that can guide future actions.

The book begins with a set of essays that provide background on various aspects of the history of medicine as well as an overview of the early women's medical movement. The second section features a chronological accounting

5

of women's entry into the American medical profession, told firsthand by six remarkable pioneering women physicians. A timeline, depicting key events in U.S. and medical history, offers context. Scattered throughout this section are contemporary quotes from participants in the nineteenth-century debate over woman's proper place.

Next, we meet the twenty members of the Class of 1879 of the Woman's Medical College of Pennsylvania, and we follow them as students and then as practitioners. Most of this class entered medical school during the nation's centennial year. Together, they represent the "typical" late-nineteenth-century woman physician. Unlike earlier and later classes, the class of 1879 did not include a black woman. The lives and contributions of nineteenth-century black women doctors have received special attention in the original essay contributed by Darlene Clark Hine.

The last section of the book documents and analyzes the reason for the decline in the number and percentage of women physicians that occurred at the end of the nineteenth century and was not stemmed until the 1950s. It concludes with an update on women physicians in 1980.

Ideas shaped the project, but it was people who made it possible. These people include hundreds of individuals—relatives of nineteenth-century women physicians, government clerks, town historians, professionals and volunteers in local historical societies and in libraries and archives big and small, and members of my own extended family. Patricia May Bass, Katie May, and the late Stacy May worked diligently to unearth information on Dr. Sarah Cohen May, my great-grandaunt and a member of the Class of 1879.

The impetus for my decision to engage in what is now called "public history" came from my mother, Jane Maguire Abram, who instilled me with respect for the public's intelligence. From my father, Morris B. Abram, I got the idea that I could do anything I wanted. From both I learned that each of us is obliged to contribute to society's well-being. I thank them.

Credit for the organization and style of this book goes to our first editor, Maura Walsh, who demonstrated great care, persistence, and good humor. The photographs were identified and collected by Jean Houck and Carol Levkov in a national search that required painstaking detective work.

The project has been generously supported by four organizational sponsors: The American Medical Women's Association, the oldest national organization of women physicians, was established in 1915. Two national presidents, doctors Lila S. Kroser and Claire M. Callan, and Executive Director Carol Davis-Grossman effectively linked the project with AMWA's vibrant network. The Medical College of Pennsylvania was founded in 1850 as the world's first regular woman's medical college. President Maurice Clifford's personal interest has been especially helpful. The New York Infirmary/Beekman Downtown Hospital, founded in 1853 by doctors Elizabeth and Emily Blackwell, was the first hospital for women run entirely by women. I thank Mary Honaker, director of development, for her warm support. New York University's Department of History, where I learned my craft, opened its public history program in 1983. Co-director Paul Mattingly's critique of my work on the Class of 1879 of the Woman's Medical College of Pennsylvania was as inspiring as it was tough. All the organizational sponsors have contributed facilities, staff, funds, networks, and personal support. I am deeply grateful.

My research began at the Archives and Special Collections on Women in Medicine at the Medical College of Pennsylvania, where Director Sandra Chaff offered early and unwavering support. With her help and with that of Jill Gates Smith and Margaret Jerrido, hundreds of records, documents, and photographs were unearthed and reproduced. Ms. Jerrido also conducted a successful far-flung search for materials on nineteenth-century black women doctors.

The exhibition staff, an enormously talented group, included Ellen J. Smith, interpretive director; Steve Brosnahan, architectural designer; Karen Smith, graphics designer; Gregg Miller, audio designer; Mary Jane Soule, sound producer, Beverly Simon, curriculum writer; and Helen Illig and Carol Levkov, administrators. Ms. Illig stuck with the project during its initial and sometimes bleak days, a vote of confidence that won't be forgotten. Ellen Smith shared responsibility for planning and executing this project. Her array of skills and her reassuring style have served us well. I have thoroughly enjoyed our partnership.

The breadth and skill of the scholars writing in this book is self-evident. I am indebted to Regina Morantz-Sanchez, who generously shared her information and encouraged me to pursue this topic. It was from Mary Roth Walsh's *Doctors Wanted: No Women Need Apply* that I first learned of the history interpreted by this project. I have referred to this groundbreaking work repeatedly.

From the beginning, the project was blessed by a stellar advisory board. Scholars, physicians, and community volunteers lent time, advice, and all manner of support. The members were Claire M. Callan, Sandra Chaff, Carol Davis-Grossman, Virginia Drachman, Darlene Clark Hine, Alan Koslow, Ross Kraemer, Virginia Kress, Lila S. Kroser, Paul Mattingly, Alice McCone, Edith Mayo, Barbara Melosh, Regina Morantz-Sanchez, Carol Nadelson, Carl Prince, Susan Reverby, Horace B. Robinson, Charles Rosenberg, Morris Vogel, and Deborah Warner.

W. W. Norton became our publisher because Jim Mairs saw a real book in the plans for the exhibit. Jeremy Townsend made it happen.

The National Endowment for the Humanities provided the financial assistance necessary to plan and then implement the project. The NEH was joined by the following contributors: Sophia Fund, H. J. Heinz Corporation, Abbott Laboratories, Pfizer Pharmaceuticals, Josiah Macy Foundation, the Susan Smith McKinney Steward Society, Inc., the Episcopal Diocese of Pennsylvania, the Medical College of Pennsylvania Alumnae Association, Mathilde and Arthur B. Krim Foundation, the Metropolitan Life Insurance Corporation, and hundreds of women doctors. Pat Carbine, publisher of *Ms.* magazine, lent her creative genius and contacts in the search for funds.

To my husband, Herbert Teitelbaum, and to my children, Anna and Noah, I offer my thanks and my love. You have given me what no one else could—a sense of personal balance and joy and the deep security of family life.

ACKNOWLEDGMENTS

Contents

Part Three

HER CALLING IN LIFE
The Class of 1879 of the Woman's Medical College of Pennsylvania

Part Four

RELAPSE/DIAGNOSIS
The Turn-of-the-Century Decline of Women Physicians

The purpose of the women's medical movement is for occupying positions which men can not fully occupy and exercising an influence which men can not wield at all.
                                                                —*Dr. Elizabeth Blackwell*

We should give to man cheerfully the curative department and women the preventive.
                                                                —*Dr. Harriet Hunt*

What men have done for the development of science, [women] will do for suffering humanity.
                                                                —*Dr. Mark Kerr*

From towns and cities, we are frequently receiving the inquiry, "Can you not send us a reliable lady physician?"
                                                                —*Dr. Ann Preston*

Part One

BETWEEN TWO WORLDS

Nineteenth-Century American Medicine

Introduction

WHEN, in the middle decades of the nineteenth century, American women commenced their march into the medical profession, that profession was in considerable disarray. Few men of good breeding and superior education selected medicine as a career, and those who did enjoyed little of the prestige and community goodwill afforded their modern counterparts.

Medical education was catch-as-catch-can, a private arrangement between a student and a practitioner, followed, sometimes, by a short stint in one of the many medical schools springing up around the countryside. These schools, both "regular" (from which modern medical schools are descended) and "irregular" (i.e., colleges of Eclectic medicine, homeopathy, and osteopathy), were regarded mainly as vehicles for the advancement of professors' pecuniary interests. In a time when effective medical therapies were few and far between, graduates of either camp competed openly and savagely for a relatively small patient population.

It is more than coincidental that the door to medical education for women opened at this time, when the medical profession was at such a low ebb. If there was one point on which most Victorians agreed, it was that women were particularly virtuous, the moral "housekeepers" of society. This community consensus on the restorative powers of "Virtuous Womanhood" provided an important basis for the argument in favor of women physicians: women would "uplift" the profession.

Throughout the nineteenth century, leaders of the women's medical movement would emphasize this point. Dr. Joseph S. Longshore, a founding trustee

15

of the Woman's Medical College of Pennsylvania, took the occasion of that institution's first commencement exercise to give the following advice to the ladies seated before him: "Those who are most interested in you and the great enterprise in which you have enlisted look to *you* to elevate the standard of the profession."[1] Dr. Ann Preston reminded the Woman's Medical College Class of 1858, "You take into the profession an element essential to its completeness . . . the spirit and life of true woman . . . and infuse a deeper reverence and purity in the ranks."[2] Women rode into the disreputable medical profession on a wave of this public belief in their special virtues.

If the presence of women was the most visible change in nineteenth-century medicine, it was by no means the only change. Indeed, as the following essays suggest, almost everything about American medicine was in flux. No story of women's entry into medicine as professional housekeepers could be complete without an understanding of the state of the house.

NOTES

1. Joseph S. Longshore, "A Valedictory Address Delivered Before the Graduating Class at the First Annual Commencement of the Female Medical College of Pennsylvania" (Philadelphia: Medical College of Pennsylvania Archives and Special Collection on Women in Medicine, 1851).
2. Ann Preston, "A Valedictory Address to the Graduating Class of the Female Medical College of Pennsylvania for the Session of 1857–1858" (Ibid., 1858).

Soon the Baby Died

Medical Training in Nineteenth-Century America

NEITHER the absence of a college education
nor the lack of a medical degree prevented anyone from practicing medicine
in nineteenth-century America. Writing in *Harper's Magazine* in 1876, the
notable nineteenth-century diagnostician Dr. Austin Flint explained, "There
are practically no legal restrictions on the practice of medicine in most States
of the Union. . . . Rarely, if ever, are legal penalties, if they exist, enforced
for practicing without a diploma or license." Therefore, concluded Flint, only
"desire for instruction" drew students to medical schools.[1] By 1880, this desire
had prompted 11,826 people to enroll in America's seventy-five medical schools.[2]

Throughout the colonial period, most people acquired medical training by
serving apprenticeships with practicing physicians. After about three years,
the students received certificates attesting to their medical abilities and good
characters. Thus armed, new "doctors" commenced their practices. Even
after medical schools were established in the United States (the first, the
University of Pennsylvania Medical School, was founded in 1765), training
at these institutions was regarded simply as a supplement to the apprenticeship
or preceptor system. Speaking in 1854, Dr. Ellwood Harvey, Professor of the
Principles and Practice of Medicine at the Woman's Medical College of Pennsylvania, spoke favorably of America's lax regulations. From Harvey's perspective, lack of regulation placed the responsibility for choosing between

17

educated and uneducated physicians where it belonged—on the public. "There can be no permanent harm," Harvey asserted, "in allowing the people to think and act and choose for themselves." A diploma from a medical school, Harvey opined, was simply "proof that [doctors] do not assume such a responsible position without adequate preparation."[3] Unfortunately, even those earnest gentlemen who did go to the trouble and expense of acquiring a medical school education had reason to doubt the adequacy of their preparation.

Easy to organize and profitable for the professors who established them, proprietary medical schools flourished in America after the War of 1812. A term of study consisted of a three- to four-month series of lectures, and students were awarded degrees after completing only two such terms, the second of which was an exact repetition of the first. Professors, who received no salary, were recompensed through the sale of admission tickets to their lectures; because larger classes meant higher incomes, large classes prevailed. By 1850, when the first women's medical school was founded, there were forty-two such schools in America, as compared with three in France.[4]

Confronted with a limited pool of applicants and aware that even unqualified students rejected by their college would most likely be welcomed with open arms by their competitors, medical educators were not particularly discriminating in their admissions policies. In the 1876 *Harper's Magazine* article mentioned earlier, Austin Flint described the dilemma most American medical schools faced throughout the nineteenth century: "A medical college can not, without risk of its prosperity, require a higher grade of preliminary study or qualification for a degree than those institutions with which it is in immediate competition."[5] Women's medical schools, however, did not suffer such competition and were thus able to maintain higher standards of education.

Actually, the "best" students rarely applied to medical schools, for medicine was not considered a prestigious field throughout most of the nineteenth century. Dr. J. Marion Sims, who went on to become one of the century's greatest gynecological surgeons, remembered that in 1832, when he told his father that he intended to go to medical school, the elder Mr. Sims objected, calling medicine a "profession for which [he had] the utmost contempt."[6] A survey conducted by the American Medical Association in 1851 simply confirmed what was common knowledge: graduates of the better colleges rarely sought training in medicine.[7]

Despite his father's objections, Marion Sims went on to obtain as fine a mid-nineteenth-century medical education as could be had in America. Not only did he serve a long apprenticeship under a practicing physician, but he completed fourteen-week courses of study at both the Charleston Medical School and Philadephia's noted Jefferson Medical College. Yet Sims, like many physicians just starting out in his day, soon discovered some gaping holes in his medical education. Toward the end of his illustrious career, Sims was fond of recounting the dreadful story of his first two patients, who came to call in 1835. "[My first] patient was a baby about eighteen months old who had what we would call the summer complaint or chronic diarrhea. I examined this child minutely from head to foot. I looked at its gums and, as I always

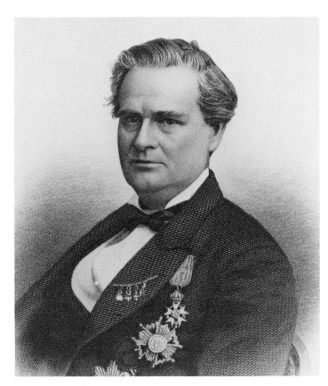

J. Marion Sims, 1813–1883 (1850s). NLM.

carried a lancet and had surgical propensities, as soon as I saw some swelling of the gums, I at once took out my lancet and cut the gums down to the teeth . . . but when it came to making up a prescription, I had no more idea what ailed the child or what to do for it than if I had never studied medicine."

Sims explained to the mother that he had to return to his office to make up a prescription, which she might call for shortly. He remembered poring over his medical "library" for a treatment: "I hurried back to my office and I took out one of my seven volumes of Eberle, which comprised my library . . . and turned to the subject of Cholera Infantum and read it through, over and over again. . . . It was my only resource. . . . At the beginning of his article . . . there was a prescription. I compounded it as quickly as I knew how and had everything in readiness for the arrival of [the mother]."

Soon the doctor received another call from the distraught mother, who explained that the prescription hadn't helped. Sims again took up his single sourcebook: "I turned to Eberle again and to a new leaf. I gave the baby a prescription from the next chapter. Suffice it to say that I changed leaves and prescriptions as often as once or twice a day. The baby continued to grow weaker." To the horror of the young physician, the baby soon died.

About a fortnight later, Sims received his second patient, a baby whose symptoms, much to the doctor's dismay, matched those of the first: "I was nonplussed. I had no authority to consult but Eberle; so I took up Eberle again, and this time I read him backwards. I thought I would reverse the treatment . . . [but] the baby got no better from the very first. And soon this baby died."[8]

The fact was, physicians of Sims's day were generally powerless against the summer complaint, from which infants died in great numbers well into the twentieth century. Only with the arrival of antibiotics and methods of intravenous feeding would doctors be able to arrest the dehydration from which these babies ultimately perished. Nevertheless, our class valedictorian's inability even to recognize this extremely common condition illustrated the failings of a completely unregulated educational system. Although late-nineteenth-century reformers, including prominent members of the women's medical movement, would lobby for national adherence to minimum educational standards, throughout most of the century freedom from regulation prevailed. Insofar as it contributed indirectly to medicine's bad reputation and encouraged the proliferation of new medical schools, this freedom was an important factor in women's midcentury entrance into the field.

Although too late for J. Marion Sims, American medical schools gradually did adopt higher standards. Harvard Medical School took the lead, largely through the efforts of Charles Eliot, who became president of Harvard University in 1869. By 1871, Harvard had done away with the lecture-ticket system and placed each professor on a salary. The academic year had expanded from four to nine months, and students were required to attend three of these expanded terms and to pass all of their final examinations in order to graduate. Although these more stringent standards caused a temporary drop in enrollment, Harvard held fast. Its decision, Eliot noted with pleasure in 1880, resulted in a markedly higher caliber of student.[9]

Strengthened and revised versions of Harvard's reforms were eventually adopted by other prestigious regular medical schools, both male and female. Although many medical schools—particularly homeopathic and Ecletic ones— would successfully resist growing pressure to conform up through the turn of the century, most late-nineteenth-century educators recognized the reforms initiated at Harvard as the wave of the future.

NOTES

1. Austin Flint, "Medical and Sanitary Progress," *Harper's New Monthly Magazine*, 53 (June 1876): 71.
2. Paul Starr, *The Social Transformation of American Medicine: The Rise of a Sovereign Profession and the Making of a Vast Industry* (New York: Basic Books, 1982), 112.
3. Ellwood Harvey, M.D., *Valedictory Address*, Female Medical College of Pennsylvania, 1854.
4. Starr, *Social Transformation*, 42.
5. Flint, "Medical and Sanitary Progress," 71.
6. Starr, *Social Transformation*, 82.
7. Ibid., 82.
8. Agnes C. Vietor, ed., *A Woman's Quest: The Life of Marie Zakrzewska, M.D.* (New York and London: Appleton Books, 1924), 274–76.
9. Starr, *Social Transformation*, 112–15.

American Medicine in 1879

CHARLES E. ROSENBERG

As the 1870s drew to a close, few thoughtful Americans could have escaped the conviction that their children would inherit a world very different from their own. The United States was a nation of almost fifty million; the census of 1870 had enumerated only thirty-nine million, an increase of roughly a quarter in the decade. America was already an economic giant. Such rapid development had left an awareness of friction and conflict—the labor violence of 1877 and the panic of 1873 were still fresh in American minds—though mixed with a lingering faith in the potential of technology, of science, of growth itself. The city and factory seemed the necessary future shape of America. The great majority of Americans, however, still lived on farms and in villages, thirty-six million in towns of less than twenty-five hundred.[1] The city embodied the future and a new style of life, but it was not yet the way of life followed by most Americans.

No sector of the American experience was changing more rapidly than that of learning and the communities of men who accumulated, disseminated, and applied it. The increasing complexity of social organization and elaboration

Reprinted with changes from "Between Two Worlds: American Medicine in 1879," from *Centennary of Index Medicus*, John Blake, ed. Maryland: National Institute of Health, 1980.

of knowledge implied the creation of new careers and new modes of coping with an ever-increasing body of information.[2] The *Index Medicus,* on the one hand, and the career of its organizer, John Shaw Billings, represent these new realities in a particularly appropriate way. But this example was hardly atypical. The American Bar Association was organized in 1878; the Johns Hopkins University, with its novel emphasis on advanced research and teaching, had opened its doors two years earlier. In that same centennial year, Thomas Edison had created America's first industrial laboratory, incorporating not only his entrepreneurial skills, but also the formal learning of European-trained scholars.[3] The intuitive tinkerer could no longer contend unaided with the complexities of a new science-based technology.

The world of medicine too was becoming complex; medical learning had to be ordered and subdued. It was already clear that no single individual could hope to master the literature of clinical medicine, let alone those rapidly expanding biological sciences that promised to become ever more closely integrated into the practice of medicine. The founding of the *Index Medicus* was no random event, but related precisely to a particular moment in social and intellectual history.

Despite such premonitions of innovation, American medicine in 1879 was still very much between two worlds, one of traditional medical practice and one of the twentieth century with its new ideas, institutions, and modes of therapeutics. Like that three-quarters of the nation's population that still lived on farms and in villages, medicine had in some ways changed little since the early nineteenth century. The average medical man still practiced much as he had in past generations. He saw patients in their homes or in his office and submitted bills to his "families" at leisurely intervals. He treated children and adults, delivered babies, lanced boils, and set broken bones. But the bulk of his therapeutics consisted, as it had for centuries, of the administration of drugs and the dissemination of reassuring words. He was far less likely, however, to bleed his patients than was his predecessor of a half-century before, and if he did employ a good number of traditional remedies, dosages were milder and the indications more carefully defined.[4] He had at his disposal, moreover, a number of new drugs and modes of administering them that promised to expand his limited therapeutic repertoire. Salicylic acid, for example, with its acknowledged efficacy in treating acute rheumatism seemed only the most promising of a number of fever-reducing drugs. (Some physicians warned, however, that these currently fashionable antifever drugs were already being used indiscriminately and with little attention to their possible dangerous side effects.) Electrotherapeutics too seemed of proven—if admittedly diffuse—worth in a variety of conditions. Sugar-coated pills and the hypodermic syringe promised in their different ways to ease the practitioner's therapeutic rounds. Perhaps most important, physicians in 1879 could congratulate themselves that their practice was increasingly in keeping with the body's natural tendency toward healing. As one older country practitioner put it, contrasting therapeutic realities of his youth with those of 1879, "The agony of a patient with a fever *then*—parched with thirst, starved with hunger, choked with crude drugs in massive doses; and his comfort *now,* present a striking contrast."[5]

But many of the physician's most efficacious remedies—opium and its derivatives, digitalis, quinine—were hardly new to the physician's medical bag. Other, and by twentieth-century standards less useful, standbys of the traditional therapeutics still played a major role in patient care. None of these was more in evidence than the omnipresent mercury; as a salve, a purge, an "alterative," and as something of a specific remedy in syphilis, it still played a central therapeutic role despite growing awareness of its toxicity. To ambitious young physicians, however, the most exciting new horizons beckoned in the area of surgery and the surgical specialities, ophthalmology, gynecology, otology, and orthopedics. Diagnosis too boasted a new and seemingly scientific precision. The thermometer and the systematic recording of temperatures had become in the previous fifteen years a normal part of clinical routine; a few of the more ambitious were already seeking correlations between pulse and temperature as they sought to define the course of ancient ills with a new precision. The physician could call as well on a variety of chemical and physical tests of the urine, and, of even greater novelty, he could use the hemocytometer in making red cell counts. The stethoscope and ophthalmoscope had, again in the past two decades only, been added to the clinical equipment of physicians outside the select company of urban specialists and teachers.[6]

In some ways, however, the existence of these new therapeutic and diagnostic tools only underscored the persistence of other realities that had changed little indeed in the first century of medicine in the United States. Perhaps most important was the physician's marketplace position. Doctors still competed for a limited number of paying cases; only a handful of well-established practitioners could rely on a secure and remunerative return from practice. Access to the profession was still essentially uncontrolled and the costs of education small. Thus the continuing medical fear of "interference"—the anxiety that each fellow practitioner might be a competitor for one's patients, that consultations might provide the occasion for a clever and unscrupulous consultant to seduce away a previously loyal family. Not a few local and state medical societies had adopted or were considering the policy of blacklisting of recalcitrant patients; those unwilling to pay their bills would have no physician to call upon. The economic pressures physicians faced could be seen as well in repeated charges of unethical business practices, the planting of self-serving newspaper accounts of triumphant operations and unexpected cures, and the endorsement by medical men of health resorts, bottled waters, and patent remedies.[7] And physicians, of course, still contended with a host of competitors who did not even style themselves physicians, the lay practitioners of a traditional domestic medicine and the pharmacists who habitually prescribed on their own authority.

In America's cities, where change had proceeded most rapidly, competition remained intense. General practitioners resented specialists and holders of hospital and dispensary physicianships, a hostility that informed a debate over so-called "charity abuse"[8] that agitated a number of urban medical societies in 1879. The Medical Society of the County of New York, for example, held a particularly intense discussion centering on the way in which patients well able to pay for care were treated gratuitously at the city's numerous hospitals and dispensaries. Many staff physicians, it was charged, in their eagerness to exploit clinical material and enlarge their own institutional privileges, thought little of the economic plight of the ordinary practitioner. New York and Philadelphia authorities on "charity organization" drew up plans to investigate and certify the "worthiness" of applicants for clinic care; many dispensaries, traditionally free, were beginning to impose a charge of ten cents per patient visit in response to such allegations of indiscriminate alms-giving. Inpatient as well as outpatient services were recipients of similar criticism. In Philadelphia, for example, critics contended that facilities were so abundant that the city tolerated an average of eleven hundred empty beds, the equivalent of five institutions the size of Pennsylvania Hospital.[9]

Lingering hostilities still marked relationships between sectarians—most prominently homeopaths—and regular physicians. Though both groups could at times ally themselves in resisting the pretensions of the untrained and the outright quack, there remained a good deal of competition for the same limited pool of paying patients.[10]

It would be a mistake, however, to overemphasize these traditional problems, for significant changes were already apparent in the institutional structure of medical practice, changes that would become increasingly important in the next two generations. If one looks not at ordinary physicians, most of whom practiced in small towns and rural areas, but at the ambitious urban elite, one can discern a pattern of medical education and practice surprisingly similar to that which was to develop in the first half of the twentieth century. It emphasized the practice of medicine in an institutional setting, specialism, systematic clinical observation, and publication. Though few paying patients (aside from the insane) were treated in a hospital setting, an increasing number of the less prosperous sought care in a hospital or dispensary. In many cases, indeed, general practitioners were happy enough to divest themselves of difficult cases with a casual referral to a convenient outpatient department; at the same time, patients began to seek care at such institutions independently. Many urban Americans had already assimilated the consumer's wisdom that it was best to seek the diagnostic skills of "the professor" or "the specialist."[11]

The careers of ambitious young physicians were involved inextricably with these urban medical institutions: in a period without formal internships and residencies, skills and reputation in the specialties could only be acquired in the outpatient or specialized wards of hospitals and dispensaries. In every major city, moreover, the teaching of clinical medicine was centered increasingly in these institutions. In 1879 the aspiring medical student could already find clinical opportunities in every major American city and in almost every important hospital. And to the city's workingmen and -women, of course, these institutions were a necessity, despite the skepticism or fear they sometimes inspired.

To medical men at the time, however, and to the historian in retrospect, the major institutional change in American medical practice was the inexorable spread of specialism. The pages of America's leading medical journals were filled disproportionately with the case reports, review articles, and clinical lectures of neurologists, orthopedic surgeons, opthalmologists, laryngologists, otologists, dermatologists, and pediatricians. With the exception of the pediatricians and orthopedic surgeons, all of these specialties boasted national associations by 1879, and most had representatives on medical school faculties, if only in adjunct positions.[12] It must be recalled, however, that most specialists still felt some reservations about thus identifying themselves; at least two of the national associations, for example, forbade members to advertise themselves as exclusive specialists. (The otological and ophthalmological societies warned members that the titles "aurist" and "oculist" could not be used in public announcements.) But such scruples did little to reassure ordinary physicians, who were threatened both by the specialists' claims to particular competence and by the willingness of many specialists to continue to serve as general practitioners and thus competitors.

Even among specialists there were occasional differences; 1879, to cite one example, marked the height of a bitter conflict between New York neurologists and leaders in the Association of Asylum Superintendents (predecessor of the American Psychiatric Association). Within the older and most prestigious hospitals, those grandees who occupied the positions of attending physician and surgeon were often unreceptive to the newer specialties. And these were not the only social differentiations that marked the profession; medicine was still essentially an occupation for white males. Though a handful of zealous and highly motivated women were able to gain medical degrees at one of America's four female medical schools (or in one of the few other less prestigious, coeducation schools), they had a difficult time in finding clinical training. Most regular medical schools would not, of course, admit blacks, nor would the American Medical Association admit black medical associations and schools to membership.[13]

Despite the often fragmented quality of the profession and the unrelenting demands of the marketplace, pressures to expand the scope of medical education increased steadily. As a supplement to training at the gradually increasing facilities for clinical education in the United States, the most ambitious and financially able sought European, and especially German, credentials. Germany had already become so fashionable that one reviewer in 1879 could note that authors would often ransack the German and English references, yet ignore equally significant work in the French literature.[14] The intellectual center of medicine had shifted drastically since those antebellum years when Paris was the goal of America's most ambitious young physicians and French was the language that provided entrée to the newest in medical ideas and techniques. Those physicians unable to afford the time or money to refine their clinical skills on the Continent would soon be able to attend intensive courses offered by newly organized postgraduate schools and polyclinics, finishing schools for those graduates who sought to update or expand their clinical skills. Despite a continuing rhetorical opposition to exclusive specialism as intellectually indefensible, it was clearly the road to success in urban practice.[15] Medical schools, not surprisingly, vied with one another in boasting of their clinical facilities and access to hospital wards and amphitheaters. New York's College of Physicians and Surgeons, for example, offered prospective students ten outpatient clinics in its own building, access to eleven of the city's hospitals and dispensaries, as well as "personal" instruction in such clinical skills as minor surgery, physical diagnosis, normal and pathological histology, physical examination of the eye, otology, practical gynecology, and laryngoscopy and rhinoscopy.[16] The more ambitious would easily find time and money to enroll in such tutorials.

Medical education was an area of criticism and change. The better institutions, Harvard and the University of Pennsylvania, for example, had already begun to raise standards, though the number of schools in which the aspiring and poorly endowed medical student could receive a degree remained high and the number of outright diploma mills may actually have increased in the years since the Civil War. Three rather than two courses of lectures were now offered—and in a few cases demanded—by the better institutions. Fall and spring courses were generally available in addition to the regular five-month winter course, thus creating an option approximating a nine-month term. (Most schools began their regular winter course on or about October the first and ended at the beginning of March, though a few tolerated shorter terms and some provided longer ones.)[17] In addition, especially motivated students used their summer months to seek clinical clerkships in flourishing dispensaries and hospital outpatient departments. Country medical schools were fading rapidly in significance as the city's clinical opportunities made medical education an almost exclusively urban phenomenon. Examinations too were becoming gradually more demanding. At New York's Physicians and Surgeons, only seventy-two of one hundred twenty applicants for the degree received it; thirty were failed and eighteen conditioned. At Harvard the previous year, only forty-seven of seventy-two applicants were granted the doctorate. The University of Pennsylvania had just lengthened its course and was about to raise its entrance requirements for the 1880–81 session.[18] The specialties, as we have noted previously, were making their way inexorably into the curriculum, as they already had into practice and into dispensary and outpatient staffs. At Chicago's Rush Medical College, for example, chairs in dermatology and orthopedic surgery were created for the first time in 1879, and gynecology and obstetrics were divided into separate positions.[19] Medical school graduates competed with increasing intensity for the limited number of hospital resident physicianships; and though it is easy to dwell on the personal and political connections that too often led to such appointments, it must be remembered that at least some were determined by competitive examination and that the number of such protointernships increased steadily.

One could, indeed, demonstrate that all of those reformist ideas that we associate with medical education in the twentieth century were already being articulated by dissatisfied spokesmen for improved standards a century ago. A "Report on Medical Education" for example, presented to the Illinois State Medical Society in 1879 contended that physicians could hardly hope to improve their economic or social status without a thorough overhauling of American medical education. Higher entrance requirements, a three-year graded term, chairs endowed so that their occupants would not be dependent on the fees of matriculants and graduates, final examination by a board unconnected with the faculty—all these were needed if ever-increasing numbers of American medical men were not to clutter a marketplace already crowded with far too many ill-trained practitioners. It was this oversupply, the report reasoned with some humor, not some perversity among their clients, that dictated the inevitable poverty of most American physicians:

> The people who inhabit the banks of the Ganges are said to rid themselves of overcrowded numbers by drowning them in its waters. Society disposes of many of the multitudinous progeny annually cast upon it from the fruitful matrices of our numerous medical schools, after short gestations and easy deliveries, by the more slow and painful process of starvation.

Most contemporaries similarly assumed a connection between the physician's market position and the system that educated him. But such material calculations were not the only motive to reform; the ideals of intellectual achievement had already been assimilated in the American medical elite. This same Illinois report also urged that the nation's medical schools "be endowed, so that their teachers might have leisure and opportunity for research, and be able to develop, as well as impart knowledge."[20] The pursuit of knowledge, status, and dollars seemed nicely consistent.

But such ideas were not, of course, to become the basis of a uniform policy before the twentieth century. Most American medical schools were in no position to take advantage of such admonitions, and their students were ill-prepared financially and intellectually for this new world of medical learning. Such realities are easily demonstrated. In the spring of 1879, a special convention of the American Medical College Association (founded only three years before) met and resolved after some debate to propose that all its member institutions raise their entrance requirements and institute a three-year program. These brave resolves were quickly tabled, however, when the association itself met in regular session.[21] Most schools simply could not afford to incur such a competitive disadvantage in their never-ending search for crowded classrooms.

For the first time, at least some of the states were considering more rigid licensing. In 1879, however, Illinois was the only state with an examination and licensing system approximating that of the twentieth century. And though still opposed by some practitioners within the state, the system did seem to be having an effect. Medical editorialists were pleased to note that after only a year of effective operation, Illinois had rid itself of roughly fifteen hundred unqualified practitioners—many of whom had moved to nearby states.[22] Based on a coalition of homeopathic, eclectic, and regular support and board membership, the Illinois licensing body seemed to many physicians a model of political astuteness. But the Illinois solution was clearly atypical. In most states and most areas of potential medical policy, the role of government was slight indeed.

Only in public health did there seem to be an awakening sense of state and even national responsibility. In every urban area, discussion of tenement house conditions and environmental sanitation had become commonplace, even if reform efforts often proved abortive. Following the lead of Massachusetts in 1869, moreover, state after state had moved to create boards of health; by 1879 twenty such health boards had come into existence (though in some states that existence was fragile indeed).[23] Moreover, the most dramatic medical event of 1879 was to take place in the sphere of public medicine. In the wake of a traumatic yellow fever epidemic that had scarred the Mississippi Valley in the previous year, Congress created a precedent-setting National Board of Health. Physicians were unable to agree upon yellow fever's cause and mode of transmission, but they could agree that national quarantine was a practical necessity. Though now researchers suppose that local environmental factors might play a role in fostering the disease, few medical men then doubted that yellow fever was often if not invariably introduced by ships from tropical ports.[24] Although the National Board was to survive bureaucratic infighting and federal passivity only a half-dozen years, it did constitute a concrete recognition of the growing conviction that in some areas at least the federal government should exert a necessary and truly national authority. Yellow fever, ironically still a mystery to the world of scientific medicine, had served as a crystallizing force in encouraging public recognition of medicine's scientific claims.

Perhaps most fundamental to medical thought was the evolving complex of ideas surrounding disease. Though educated physicians had become accustomed to thinking of the most important infectious ills as specific, much confusion remained. Many physicians, for example, still found it natural to believe that one disease could transform itself into another and that undesirable environmental conditions could—of themselves—breed sickness. Sewer gas, for example, was still highly suspect as a cause of diphtheria, typhoid fever, and surgical infection. The relationship between a number of seemingly distinct ills remained unclear; the possible identities of croup and diphtheria, for example, were widely discussed in 1879, as was the existence of an elusive typhomalarial fever. Similarly, the clinical course of a specific nature of syphilis remained an area of conjecture. Especially in such constitutional ills as tuberculosis and rheumatism, physicians still emphasized questions of heredity and predisposition, and in so doing reaffirmed in appropriately modern guise the traditional categories of humoral medicine.[25] Physicians still clung to older holistic views of causation, etiologies based on the relationship between internal and external environment, between endowment and experience. The reductionist assumption that a specific organism might be responsible for the manifestation of a particular disease seemed difficult to comprehend; though there was much talk of a "germ theory," it was enveloped in obscurity and was received with incomprehension and hostility.

It must be recalled that the constancy and variety of bacterial species was still a matter of speculation, as was the relationship between the presence of microorganisms in a suppurating lesion or disease state and their possible causative role. Only a small minority of physicians committed themselves to the concept of an exclusive role for bacteria in the causation of particular ills; for most constitutional ailments, however, this was not considered even a possible explanation. There certainly was some acknowledgement of a "contagious principle" at work in the spread of infectious ills, but its nature remained obscure. As the editor of New York's widely read *Medical Record* put it,

We can say, with much positiveness, to be sure, that it is no visible form of bacterium or micrococcus, and we can, perhaps, infer from analogy that it is a particulate something too small to be detected by the microscope, that it is albuminoid in composition and multiplies at the expense of physiological processes. Whether it is living or dead, whether it is the degenerated protoplasm of man or the modified protoplasm of vegetable, whether it acts in conjunction with bacteria or feeds directly upon the tissues, all these questions are much beyond the pathologist as yet.[26]

To most physicians this was an area of academic speculation and only marginally a matter of immediate concern.

It was in surgery that the discussion of infection was most pressing. Questions of everyday procedure were necessarily involved, questions dramatically and unavoidably crystallized in the name and ideas of Joseph Lister. No surgeon could avoid taking a position on Lister and antisepsis. What is surprising among American surgeons in 1879 is the comparatively small amount of opposition to what was called antiseptic surgery, though definitions, of course, varied widely. Many physicians adopted some version of Lister's procedures, including the much-vexed carbolic acid spray. Several, however, did not understand or accept the underlying Listerian assumption that even one organism might be the cause of a possibly fatal wound infection. Some surgeons still argued that antisepsis meant nothing more than systematic cleanliness and balked at the practical difficulties of using Lister's dressings, mode of drainage, and, of course, the carbolic spray. Some continued to emphasize as well the importance of the patient's vitality and state of nutrition to a successful surgical outcome, as well as the efficacy of particular drugs or procedures in combating shock.

In some ways it could be argued that the acceptance of Listerism was based to an extent on an apparent consistency with certain older ideas; the spray, for example, represented a practical and conceptual continuity with far older emphases on the role of the atmosphere in causing wound infection. (Medical men in 1879 still discussed instances in which sewer gas or ill-placed drains had contaminated a hospital's atmosphere and thus caused fevers and infections; it is not surprising that proper siting and ventilation were seen as remedies for such ills.) The germ theory too seemed consistent with certain older explanations of wound infection, with ideas of contamination and subsequent putrefactive change.[27] Perhaps the most fundamental basis for surgical interest in Lister and his doctrines lay, as I have suggested, in their relevance to everyday procedures. His views were not simply a matter for pathological speculation because they were expressed as specific recommendations about choice of dressings, mode of drainage, and use of carbolized silk for sutures. Most of internal medicine, by contrast, could be carried on in traditional fashion. Isolating the cause of epidemic ills seemed a far less pressing need then discovering plausible therapeutics in internal medicine. And here the germ theory seemed at best potentially relevant.

It is significant, moreover, that with the exception of the role of Pasteur and early bacteriology in the formulation of Lister's own ideas, the immediate impact of the biological sciences on clinical medicine was still slight. Even the most intellectually exacting of the clinical journals found little space in their pages for articles on the laboratory sciences, even in the sections devoted to abstracts. The great majority of the journal literature still consisted of case reports (albeit increasingly in the specialties), essays of clinical reflection and speculation, and transcriptions of clinical lectures at the nation's leading hospitals and medical schools. "Practical" and "experienced" were repeated again and again as terms of reassurance in book reviews, whereas the term "theoretical" played a symmetrically pejorative role. Even in Germany, of course, most physicians devoted themselves to clinical work and insofar as they published, did so in clinical medicine. In the United States, however, the balance of effort seemed markedly skewed toward the practical and clinical. A bibliography of publications in physiology for 1879 published by the British *Journal of Physiology,* for example, showed 59 monographs and 500 articles in German, 17 monographs and 227 articles in French—and only 2 monographs and 24 articles by American authors. If one considers the total number of articles in *Index Medicus* for that year, however, the results are quite different. Of more than 20,000 articles indexed, 4,781 were of American authorship, 4,608 French, and 4,027 German.[28]

In the minds of many Americans, indeed, there seemed to be a fundamental inconsistency between the demands of the laboratory and those of the bedside. When eulogizing J. B. S. Jackson, the prominent Boston pathologist who died in 1879, Oliver Wendell Holmes made it clear that he felt Jackson's analytical and intellectually meticulous manner made him an unsuccessful practitioner. "He was perhaps too sensitive," Holmes explained, "and, if such a word may be ventured, too scrupulous. . . . Perhaps he knew too much; knew the tricks of nature which baffle the most skillful diagnosticians too well to speak with that positiveness which is often decisive, in virtue of its personal emphasis, in cases where doubts are plenty and convictions feeble."[29] The practitioner, Holmes conceded, had to act with an entire, if necessarily arbitrary, confidence—an attitude entirely unsuitable to the scientist. Holmes was obviously aware as well that few, if any, medical men could hope to live the scientist's intellectually austere life; America in 1879 would not support them.

Contemporaries, nevertheless, were well aware that they lived in an age of change, that medicine particularly was very much in transition, and that the chief agent of change would be the very science that, for the moment at least, played so marginal a role in the average physician's practice. In his eulogy of Jackson, to pursue the same example, Holmes made it clear that his deceased friend's pathology was in its content already out of date; Jackson's gross pathology had already been superseded by that of a new generation of microscopic histologists with research rooted in skills the older man had never mastered.[30]

This self-conscious mood of transition is exemplified equally well in contemporary reactions to other deaths in 1879, the end of lives both real and at the same time symbolic of fundamental change in American medicine. Among such worthies were George Bacon Wood and Isaac Hays in Philadelphia, and Jacob Bigelow as well as Jackson in Boston. Born in 1796, Hays had edited the *American Journal of the Medical Sciences* for a half century; he had nurtured the fledgling journal into an internationally recognized quarterly from whose pages—as Hays's admirers contended—the medical progress of a half century could be reconstructed. George B. Wood (author both of an extremely successful textbook of medicine and, with Franklin Bache, of the first comprehensive *United States Dispensatory*, published in 1833, which had gone through six editions and sold well over one hundred thousand copies by 1879) was a prototype of the library scholar, the master of an already extensive clinical literature, but a stranger to the laboratory. No successor could hope to match Wood's synoptic knowledge of the medical literature; by 1879 the scope of medical literature had already become too broad. Jacob Bigelow was also mourned in 1879. Born in 1787, Bigelow's life encompassed almost a century of ever-more-rapid medical change. Bigelow's youthful publications in botany and technology illustrate the broad intellectual interests and diffuse career patterns of early-nineteenth-century physicians, while his central role in attacking the needlessly complex prescriptions and heroic dosages of the 1820s and 1830s underscores another central development in American medicine during the middle third of the nineteenth century.[31] One can, in short, cite any number of indicators of the changed yet peculiarly transitional quality of American medicine in 1879.

Medical publishing itself is a particularly relevant indicator of change, relevant certainly to our present concerns. It is no accident that the *Index Medicus* appeared in 1879. Its existence reflected a genuine need for control of an enormously varied and daily-increasing literature. The *Index* surveyed more than five hundred journal titles and cited more than twenty thousand references. In its first issue, significantly, John Shaw Billings explained why he had dismissed the possibility of issuing this new tool as an annual; knowledge was changing too rapidly, he contended, and a legitimate demand "to bring the stock of knowledge up to the very latest date" dictated a monthly format. At the same time, consistently, the American Medical Association's annual volume of *transactions* was being criticized as excessively dilatory in appearance; "few men of reputation," as one editor put it, "will submit to such delay."[32] No previous generation of physicians experienced such a pace of intellectual work; years, not months, would have been appropriate for an index a generation earlier, decades, not years, in previous centuries. Eighteen seventy-nine was perhaps a year of transition, of conceptual and institutional inconsistency and asymmetry, but the shape of future developments was already becoming clear.

NOTES

1. U.S. Bureau of the Census, *Historical Statistics of the United States, Colonial Times to 1970, Bicentennial Edition*, 2 pts., (Washington, D.C.: Government Printing Office, 1976), pt. 1:8, 12, 14, 19.
2. For a recent survey of scholarship in this area, see Alexandra Oleson and John Voss, eds., *The Organization of Knowledge in Modern America, 1860–1920* (Baltimore: Johns Hopkins University Press, 1979). See also Alfred D. Chandler's recent synthesis of business history, technology, and organizational structure in shaping administrative roles, *The Visible Hand: The Managerial Revolution in American Business* (Cambridge, MA: Harvard University Press, 1977).

3. See, for a general appraisal, Thomas P. Hughes, "Edison's Method," in William B. Pickett, ed., *Technology at the Turning Point* (San Francisco: San Francisco Press, 1977), 5–22.

4. For general discussions of these trends, see Charles E. Rosenberg, "The Therapeutic Revolution: Medicine, Meaning and Social Change in Nineteenth-Century America," *Perspectives in Biology and Medicine* 20 (1977): 485–506, and John Harley Warner, "The Nature Trusting Heresy: American Physicians and the Concept of the Healing Power of Nature in the 1850's and 1860's," *Perspectives in American History* 11 (1977–78): 291–324.

5. Samuel Peters (Cohoes, N.Y.) "Some Points in the Treatment of Typhoid Fever," *Medical Record* 15 (May 31, 1879): 508–9. It must be emphasized, however, that despite such brave disavowals of traditional therapeutic routinism and emphasis on the body's natural powers of recuperation in most ills, the clinical literature in 1879 indicates an almost universal use of drugs (frequently in imaginative combinations) in almost every conceivable clinical situation. This generalization and many of the other observations made in the following pages are based particularly on a reading of the *Boston Medical and Surgical Journal* and *Medical Record* for 1879 (cited hereafter *BMSJ* and *MR*).

6. Published case reports and hospital records make this evident, contrasting sharply with the situation during the Civil War years. See Charles E. Rosenberg, "The Practice of Medicine in New York a Century Ago," *Bulletin of the History of Medicine* 41 (1967): 223–53.

7. See, for example, Editorial, "Medical Certificates," *MR* 15 (May 24, 1879): 493–94, and 15 (June 21, 1879), 578–79; "Medical Reports in the Newspapers," ibid. 15 (Apr. 26, 1879): 404–5; "Collecting Doctor's Bills," ibid. 16 (Oct. 4, 1879): 312.

8. For a general discussion of the dispensaries and outpatient medicine, the target of most attacks on excessive charity, see: Charles E. Rosenberg, "Social Class and Medical Care in Nineteenth-Century America: The Rise and Fall of the Dispensary," *Journal of the History of Medicine* 29 (1974): 32–54; George Rosen, "The First Neighborhood Health Center Movement: Its Rise and Fall," *American Journal of Public Health* 61 (1971): 1620–37.

9. "Medical Notes: New York," *BMSJ* 100 (Mar. 20, 1879): 405; "Medical Notes: Philadelphia" and "Letter from Philadelphia," ibid., 100 (Jan. 2, 1879): 34–36. The Medical Society of the County of New York meeting is reported in detail in *MR* 15 (May 31, 1879): 524–27, and 15 (June 21, 1879): 586–88. See also related correspondence and editorials in ibid. 15 (June 21, 1879): 578, and 16 (July 23, 1879): 140–41.

10. In some ways, hostility was less than monolithic, certainly in the pages of the *MR* and *BMSJ*. For representative comments, see Editorial, "The American Medical Association," *MR* 15 (Apr. 26, 1879): 400; "The National Board of Health and Homeopathy," ibid. 15 (June 28, 1879): 621; 16 (Aug. 9, 1879): 142–32; *BMSJ* 100 (Jan. 23. 1879): 137.

11. See the comments of H. D. Noyes, *MR* 15 (May 31, 1879): 524–25.

12. Most of these specialty societies had been established in the 1870s, with the exception of asylum superintendents (1844), opthalmologists (1864), and otologists (1868). For general discussions of the rise of specialization, see George Rosen, *The Specialization of Medicine, with Particular Reference to Ophthalmology* (New York: Froben Press, 1944); Rosemary Stevens, *American Medicine and the Public Interest* (New Haven, CT: Yale University Press, 1971), 34–54.

13. Mary Roth Walsh, *"Doctors Wanted: No Women Need Apply": Sexual Barriers in the Medical Profession, 1835–1975* (New Haven, CT: Yale University Press,

1977); W. Montague Cobb, *The First Negro Medical Society: A History of the Medico-Chirurgical Society of the District of Columbia, 1884–1939* (Washington, D.C.: Associated Publisher, 1939).

14. *BMSJ* 100 (Jan. 23, 1879): 125.

15. Such formal objections to specialism hinged on the presumed inability of the exclusive specialist to deal with the body as an integrated whole.

16. College of Physicians and Surgeons, New York, *Annual Catalogue and Announcement* (New York, 1879): 17–20. These offerings were more varied than most, but all urban schools provided such alluring lists of clinical facilities, although students often discovered that reality did not entirely correspond to such expansive descriptions. For a general introduction to the problem, see Dale C. Smith, "The Emergence of Organized Clinical Instruction in the Nineteenth-Century American Cities of Boston, New York and Philadelphia" (Ph.D. diss., University of Minnesota, 1979).

17. There was no consistency as to length of term. Those schools providing an optional third year often lowered fees for those undertaking it.

18. *MR* 15 (June 7, 1879): 551; *BMSJ* 100 (Mar. 13, 1879): 373.

19. *MR* 15 (Mar. 22, 1879): 287; *BMSJ* 100 (Mar. 20, 1879): 406–7.

20. E. Ingals et al., "Report on Medical Education," *Transactions of Anniversary Meeting of the Illinois State Medical Society* 29 (1879): 228–40 (quotations pp. 233 and 236). For a forceful parallel statement of this position, see Alfred Mercer, "Abstract of an Address on Medical Education," *BMSJ* 100 (Mar. 27, 1879): 417–26. Mercer taught at Syracuse, which, like its neighbor Albany, had adopted the three-year term.

21. *BMSJ* 100 (May 15, 1879): 680–81.

22. "Illinois State Examinations," *BMSJ* 100 (Jan. 30, 1879): 164; "The Medical Practice Act in Illinois," ibid. 100 (Feb. 20, 1879): 270; H. O. Johnson, "The Regulation of Medical Practice by State Boards of Health, as Exemplified by the Execution of the Law in Illinois," *Transactions of the American Medical Association* 30 (1879): 293–98. The same volume of the AMA *Transactions* contains an extremely useful survey of the various state societies and their powers by Stanford E. Chaille, "State Medicine and State Medical Societies": 299–355.

23. Editorial, "The Growth of State Medicine," *MR* 16 (Oct. 4, 1879): 328–29; "State Boards of Health," ibid. 15 (Mar. 22, 1879): 278.

24. *BMSJ* 100 (May 22, 1879): 715–16. The controversial literature on the cause of yellow fever and appropriate means of prevention was particularly abundant in 1878 and 1879.

26. In evaluating a monograph on gout and rheumatism, *MR*'s reviewer dismissed the author's speculative pathology by noting, "This idea cannot be considered strikingly new. Indeed, whatever be the refinements in the pathology of gout, the main idea can always be expressed broadly in the humoralistic terms of Syndeham, who says: 'The quitting of bodily exercise of a sudden causes the excrementitious part of the juices, which was formerly expelled by means of such exercise, to lie concealed in the vessels and feed the disease.' " *MR* 16 (Aug. 2, 1879): 109. See the parallel speculations of Alfred Stille on acute rheumatism, ibid. 15 (Jan. 4, 1879): 31–32. On syphilis, see Fessenden N. Otis, "Clinical Lectures on the Physiological Pathology of Syphilis. Delivered at the College of Physicians and Surgeons, New York, Session of 1878–79," *BMSJ* 100 (Feb. 13, 1879): 213–21, esp. 213–15.

26. Editorial, "The Prophylaxis of Scarlet Fever," *MR* 15 (Mar. 22, 1879): 277. George Shrady, editor of *MR,* was in other moods even more skeptical in his attitude toward the germ theory. "Judging the future by the past," he chided, "we are

likely to be as much ridiculed in the next century for our blind belief in the power of unseen germs, as our forefathers were for their faith in the influence of spirits, of certain planets, and the like, in inducing certain maladies," "The Causes of Disease," *MR* 16 (Aug. 2, 1879): 107.

27. For a more extended discussion of some aspects of this elusive question, see Charles E. Rosenberg, "Florence Nightingale on Contagion: The Hospital as Moral Universe," in idem, ed., *Healing and History: Essays for George Rosen* (New York: Neale Watson, 1979), 116–36. See also Margaret Pelling, *Cholera, Fever and English Medicine, 1825–1865* (Oxford: Oxford University Press, 1978).

28. John Shaw Billings, "Our Medical Literature," in Frank B. Rogers, ed., *Selected Papers of John Shaw Billings* (Baltimore: Medical Library Association, 1965), 117–20. Billings, like many of his elite contemporaries in 1879, was dismayed at the generally undistinguished, if abundant, quality of American medical journals. Billings, "The Medical Journals of the United States," *BMSJ* 100 (Jan. 2, 1879): 1–2; Editorial, "The Tidal Wave," ibid. 100 (Jan. 2, 1879): 30–31; "Worthless Periodicals," ibid. 100 (Feb. 27, 1879): 304–5.

29. "John Barnard Swett Jackson," *BMSJ* 100 (Jan. 9, 1879): 63–64. It might be noted in passing that William Henry Welch was admitted to fellowship in the New York Academy of Medicine on May 1, 1879.

30. Ibid., p. 64. Two other eulogists, George Cheever and H. I. Bowditch, made the same point in regard to Jackson. *BMSJ* 100 (Feb. 6, 1879): 190–91.

31. See the memorial remarks of H. I. Bowditch at a meeting of the Boston Society for Medical Improvement, *BMSJ* 100 (Feb. 6, 1879): 193–95, and remarks at Suffolk District Medical Society, ibid. 100 (Mar. 27, 1879): 436–37.

32. Ibid. 100 (May 1, 1879): 614–15. Billing's comment is to be found on p. 3 of the first number of *Index Medicus*.

Tools of the Trade

Late-Nineteenth-Century Medical Instruments

ALAN R. KOSLOW

MEDICINE in the 1880s was just beginning to enter the physiological era, when for the first time physicians became interested in measuring and documenting such indicators of health as body temperature, pulse, and blood pressure. These and other physiological parameters were monitored and recorded with scrupulous precision, if not with complete understanding, and designers of medical instruments were hard-pressed to meet the demands of a newly scientific medical market.

Aside from the stethoscope, the most common and easily recognized medical "instrument" is the doctor's black bag. In point of fact, however, the "black bag" of the late nineteenth century was not always black and not always a bag. Ever-creative medical supply companies produced a variety of colors and styles to suit the different needs of individual physicians.

The bag shown here was carried by a nonsurgical, urban doctor of the late nineteenth century and contained an assortment of pharmaceutical agents for both oral and nonoral administration; diagnostic tools such as tongue depressors, a nasal speculum, a stethoscope, and an indirect laryngoscope; and some therapeutic articles such as lances and probes—a characteristic mix of old and new tools of the trade.

A traveling surgeon of the same era, however, would have carried a different sort of bag. If he was among the enlightened majority of doctors who

35

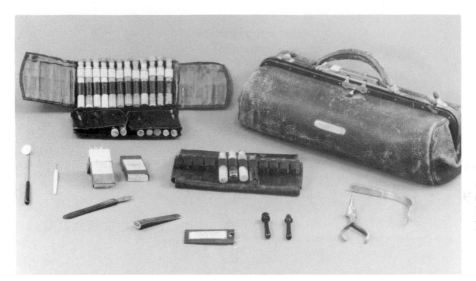

Doctor's bag (late nineteenth century). Lane Medical Library, Stanford University Medical Center.

recognized the importance of sterilizing surgical instruments before every use, he would have benefited from the model that contained in its bottom compartment a removable copper pan, which was filled with water and placed on folding legs over a flame. Used instruments were placed in the tray, covered, and sterilized in the pan's boiling water. After the surgical procedure, they were stowed away in the upper compartment of the bag, which also contained standard diagnostic equipment.

The rural or frontier physician did a lot of traveling on horseback, a mode of transportation for which the modified saddle bag was especially appropriate. Its two linked pouches could be slung over a horse or strapped together and carried as a suitcase. This particular example belonged to Dr. Clinton Cushing, who taught at San Francisco's Cooper Medical College in the nineteenth century. As long as doctors relied upon horses to carry them to sick beds, this bag remained popular. Another advantage of this variety of satchel was its size. It could carry an amazingly large number of instruments, including cumbersome lighting implements. The pronged candle holder on the left was wedged into a wooden wall according to the doctor's lighting needs. The hand-held, tubular candle holder on the right afforded the physician even more controlled illumination.

A smaller type of traveling case was popularized by the military surgeon of the Civil War. These cases contained assortments of surgical instruments ranging from four to ten in number. Of course, Civil War surgeons were not yet aware that sterilization of instruments between patients was a crucial factor in preventing surgical infection, and after a busy round of amputations and bullet extractions, used instruments were simply secured in rolled leather cases, jammed into pockets, and transported to the next battlefield. Needless to say, the death rate from infection among Civil War wounded was fearsomely high.

Whatever style of bag the physician carried into the last quarter of the nineteenth century, a thermometer was likely to be inside it. This remarkably

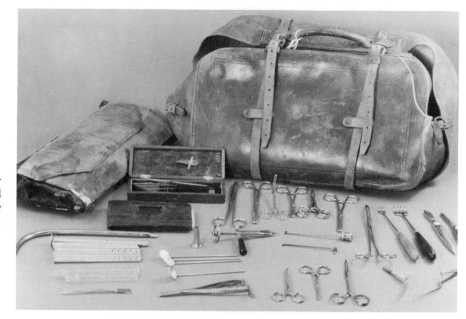

Doctor's saddlebag (late nine-teenth century). Lane Medical Library, Stanford University Medical Center.

simple instrument was first introduced in the seventeenth century, but it was the eighteenth-century clinician Hermann Boerhaave who, in consultation with G. D. Fahrenheit, standardized and refined it. There still remained the problem that the mercury reading on the thermometer would begin to fall as soon as the instrument was removed from the body orifacc. This required the physician to read the thermometer while it was still in the patient, a task both a little distasteful and so difficult that the physician needed to take the reading himself. The late-nineteenth-century physician, however, practiced in an age blessed with a truly useful refinement of clinical thermometry, the self-registering thermometer.

The self-registering thermometer helped bring the practice of medicine into the scientific era. This easy-to-use, relatively accurate instrument was a vast improvement over its predecessor. The doctor could now remove the ther-mometer from the patient with confidence that the recorded temperature would be readable until shaken down. This gave him or her the option of leaving several thermometers with the patient's family, with instructions that the temperature be taken at various times during the day. The doctor could then go about his daily rounds and still reap the diagnostic benefit of having quantified his patient's fever pattern.

It was increasingly understood that different febrile diseases followed dif-ferent fever patterns. Thus the self-registering thermometer was an invaluable aid in diagnosing these ailments. And although physicians of the day often lacked the therapeutic wherewithal to successfully treat a disease, they were nevertheless expected to be able to diagnose it and prognosticate its course. Tuberculosis, yellow and malarial fevers, and diphtheria all became readily diagnosable with the advent of the self-registering thermometer. It also gave physicians the means to test the effectiveness of treatments and, finally, to warn families of a patient's impending death. Thus the self-registering ther-

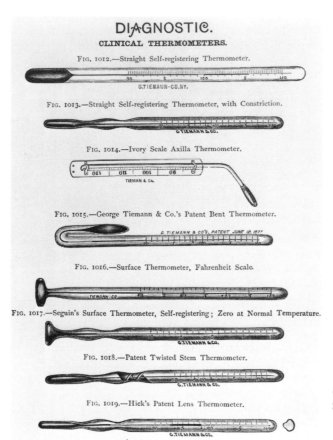

DIAGNOSTIC.
CLINICAL THERMOMETERS.
FIG. 1012.—Straight Self-registering Thermometer.
G.TIEMANN-CO.NY.
FIG. 1013.—Straight Self-registering Thermometer, with Constriction.
G.TIEMANN & CO.
FIG. 1014.—Ivory Scale Axilla Thermometer.
TIEMAN & CO.
FIG. 1015.—George Tiemann & Co.'s Patent Bent Thermometer.
G. TIEMANN & CO'S. PATENT JUNE 12, 1877
FIG. 1016.—Surface Thermometer, Fahrenheit Scale.
TIEMANN CO
FIG. 1017.—Seguin's Surface Thermometer, Self-registering; Zero at Normal Temperature.
G.TIEMANN & CO.
FIG. 1018.—Patent Twisted Stem Thermometer.
G.TIEMANN & CO.
FIG. 1019.—Hick's Patent Lens Thermometer.
G.TIEMANN & CO.
Directions for Using Thermometers.

Clinical thermometers (1889). Lane Medical Library, Stanford University Medical Center.

mometer had the dual effects of giving practitioners a needed boost in diagnostic respectability and of edging the practice of medicine into the scientific era.

Another physiological characteristic studied by late-nineteenth-century doctors was pulse. Since the time of the classical Greeks, man has known that pulse is an important indicator of health. For centuries both Western and oriental healers sought to understand what pulse rate, strength, rhythm, and regularity could reveal about disease states. The second hand on a watch was developed in the eighteenth century to serve the needs of pulse-taking physicians, and for almost fifty years, doctors were the only people who wore these unusual timepieces.

The Marey sphygmograph invented in 1860, was the first clinically useful instrument for measuring pulse. This clever device produced a graphic record of the pulse wave form, which in turn enabled the physician to quantify pulse rate, regularity, and volume, the rate of increase of the pulse form, and the rate of decrease of the pulse form. Changes in pulse could now be correlated with such clinical disease states as cardiac arrhythmias, cardiac failure, exsanguination (loss of blood), and sepsis (infection). Physicians could also use the pulse records to gauge the patient's response to treatment. Thus the sphyg-

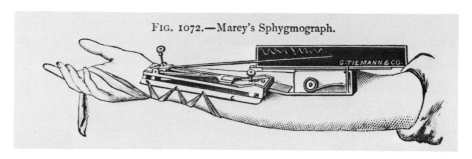

Marey's sphygmograph (1889), from the George Tiemann medical instrument catalogue. Lane Medical Library, Stanford University Medical Center.

FIG. 1072.—Marey's Sphygmograph.

mograph greatly improved the clinical abilities of the physicians who used them. The scarcity of sphygmographs in collections of antique medical instruments today, however, suggests that they were not as widely used as one might think. Whether or not this was the case, they significantly broadened our understanding of normal physiology and of many pathophysiological conditions. The new avenues of scientific endeavor stimulated by the sphygmograph eventually led to the development of such twentieth-century technological breakthroughs as the electrocardiogram.

The ophthalmoscope was yet another scientific tool that came into prominence in the last quarter of the nineteenth century. Whereas the thermometer and sphygmograph converted physiological characteristics (temperature and pulse) into statistical measures, the ophthalmoscope, with its direct view of the base of the eye, afforded physicians a direct look at internal pathology. Within a short time of its introduction in the 1860s, clinicians realized that ailments such as tumors, syphilis, Bright's disease, acute tuberculosis, locomotor ataxia, diabetes, and cerebral embolism could be indicated through a careful fundascopic examination.

The George Tiemann medical instrument catalogue of 1889 included a ten-page description of the proper uses of the ophthalmoscope, and medical journals of the day were full of positive reports about this easy-to-use diagnostic aid. Perhaps the best evidence of the ophthalmoscope's swift acceptance and widespread use, however, is the abundant number of these medical antiques still existing today. Most collections of late-nineteenth-century medical instruments used in private practice include an ophthalmoscope.

The area of medical practice that perhaps best illustrates the mix of modern and archaic therapies that characterized late-nineteenth-century medicine is obstetrics. Ignaz Semmelweis's pioneering research on puerperal fever, or child-bed fever, as it was commonly known, had vastly reduced mortality rates from infection after childbirth. But in these "dark ages" before cesarean sections became viable, physicians attending difficult deliveries were frequently forced to perform fetal craniotomies, sacrificing the infant in order to save the mother.

Before resorting to this gruesome procedure, however, late-nineteenth-century physicians brought nearly a century of refinements on obstetrical forceps to bear on the situation. Obstetricians and midwives used these simple devices to maneuver infants through the birth canal, saving countless numbers of them. Although one 1879 medical instrument catalogue offered no fewer than fifty-three varieties of this invaluable therapeutic tool, a review of in-

TOOLS OF THE TRADE

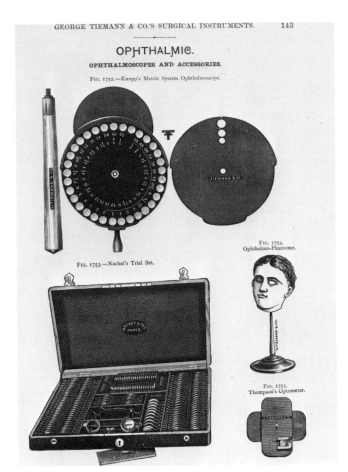

OPHTHALMIC.

OPHTHALMOSCOPES AND ACCESSORIES.

FIG. 1752.—Knapp's Metric System Ophthalmoscope.

FIG. 1753.—Nachet's Trial Set.

FIG. 1754.
Ophthalmo-Phantome.

FIG. 1755.
Thompson's Optometer.

Ophthalmoscope (1889). Lane Medical Library, Stanford University Medical Center.

strument sets in the Stanford University Medical Center collection suggests that most physicians made do with only one forcep. Hospital-based, full-time obstetricians, however had at their disposal a wide range of forceps specially designed to meet the needs of the minute. Although forceps were very successful, they were not foolproof. When the fetus's head was simply too large to fit through the birth canal, no amount of manipulation would deliver the baby.

It was in these cases of cranio-pelvic disproportionation that some of the most dreadful instruments in all of medical history were used. The 1889 George Tiemann medical instrument catalogue described their use in horrible detail:

In such instances [of imminent danger to the mother] we can still save the mother's life by sacrificing the life of her progeny. For by opening the head of the infant by means of perforating instruments, we can remove the contents of the cranium, and then break down the vault of the skull itself, and bring away the fragments piece meal, until only the base of the cranium and the bones of the face remain to be extracted by means of crotchets and other instruments.

The catalogue went on to list thirty-seven different instruments for this procedure. The collections of obstetric instruments at Stanford contained roughly five craniotomy instruments for each forcep, an indication that fetal craniotomies were performed with some frequency. Thankfully, however, surgical expertise would soon improve to the point that both mother and infant could be saved in such cases through cesarean sections.

Two developments contributed significantly to this advance in surgical therapy. First, anaesthesia was introduced in the 1840s, leading to painless surgery. Second, Joseph Lister's procedures for antiseptic surgery, which greatly reduced the risk of infection, were made known in America in the 1860s.

With the advent of painless surgery, doctors no longer needed to wait until the patient was either moribund or in such pain that any amount of surgical pain was acceptable. This new option of early surgical intervention gave many patients increased chances for survival, but the real advance that anaesthesia prompted was a rapid series of discoveries of new surgical procedures. Before anaesthesia, surgeons had to rush through operations in order to spare patients prolonged agony; anaesthesia gave physicians the time for finesse and ex-

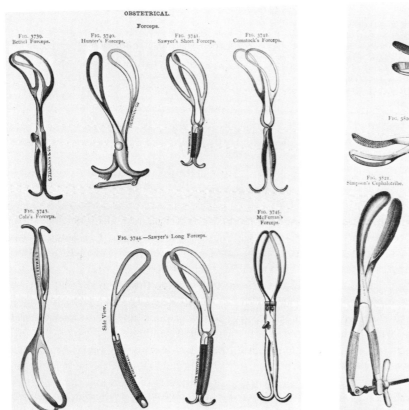
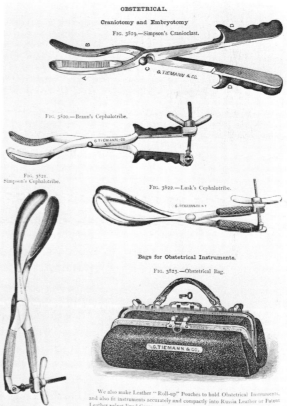

Left: *Obstetrical forceps (1889)*. Lane Medical Library, Stanford University Medical Center. Right: *Craniotomy and embryotomy instruments (1889)*. Lane Medical Library, Stanford University Medical Center.

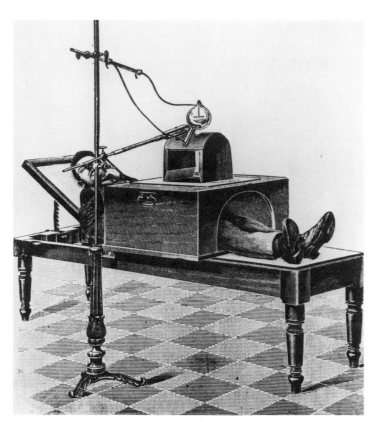

Early x-ray therapy (1890s). New York Infirmary/Beekman Downtown Hospital.

perimentation. Abdominal surgery, for example, became possible only with the arrival of ether. From the 1840s through the 1860s, previously "incurable" conditions were regularly corrected through surgery. Unfortunately, "cured" postoperative patients were dying from surgical infection with comparable regularity.

Lister's 1865 recommendations for antiseptic surgery brought infection under control. His procedures—including hand washing, disinfecting surgical instruments, and spraying disinfectant in the air around the wound—were designed to prevent bacteria from entering the surgical field. By the 1880s, most doctors followed at least some of these procedures, and the turn of the century brought universal acceptance of both the theory and practice of antiseptic surgery. These new weapons against the age-old evils of pain and infection launched the field of surgery into an era of unprecedented progress.

Thus, the late-nineteenth-century physician practiced at a pivotal point in the history of medicine. A new scientific era was dawning, shedding light on ancient mysteries in such fields as physiology, bacteriology, pathology, and pharmacology. New medical instruments and surgical procedures were being developed at an amazing pace. At the same time, however, such crude and archaic medical practices as blood letting, fetal craniotomy, and cupping lingered in the therapeutic arsenal. It was up to each individual doctor to make the difficult choices between the old and the new, but always to treat his or her patients with compassion.

Do-It-Yourself the Sectarian Way

RONALD L. NUMBERS

Among the most ardent American champions of home health care were the medical sectarians who arose in the nineteenth century to challenge the heroic therapy of the regulars with their seemingly endless rounds of bleedings, blisterings, and purgings. Over the years a multitude of sects appeared, each offering the long-suffering public a surer, safer, and often cheaper way to health. There were botanics and Eclectics, homeopaths and hydropaths, movement-curists and mind-curists, and others too numerous to mention. Despite their many differences, they all shared one trait: an enthusiasm for the practice of domestic medicine. Why they felt this way and how they related their domestic activities to other professional goals are the questions on which I shall focus. In doing so, I shall look at three of the largest and most influential of the nineteenth-century sects: the Thomsonians, the homeopaths, and the hydropaths.

While many nineteenth-century domestic medicine books fall under the general heading "botanic," the line between botanic and regular, sectarian

Reprinted, with changes, from *Medicine Without Doctors: Home Health Care in American History,* G. B. Risse, R. L. Numbers, and J. W. Leavitt, eds. (New York: Science History Publications/U.S.A., a division of Neale Watson Academic Publications, Inc., 1977), 49–72. Reprinted by permission of the author and publisher.

and nonsectarian, is often blurred.[1] John Gunn's best-selling *Domestic Medicine,* for example, contains "descriptions of the Medicinal Roots and Herbs of the United States, and how they are to be used in the cure of disease"; yet its tolerance of calomel and bleeding betrays its orthodox origins.[2] Other works on vegetable and Indian medicines were exclusively botanical, but could hardly be called sectarian in the sense of belonging to an exclusive school of medical practice.

The person who turned the root-and-herb tradition into a full-blown medical sect was Samuel Thomson, a New Hampshire farmer who learned much of his botanic medicine at the side of a local female herbalist.[3] Early in his healing career he became convinced that the cause of all disease was cold and that the only cure was the restoration of the body's natural heat. This he accomplished by steaming, peppering, and puking his patients, with heavy reliance on *lobelia,* an emetic long used by native Americans.[4]

The simplicity of his system made it ideal for domestic use. Not one to ignore the commercial possibilities of his discovery, Thomson in 1806 began selling "Family Rights" to his practice, for which he obtained a patent in 1813. For twenty dollars purchasers enrolled in the Friendly Botanic Society and received a sixteen-page instruction booklet, *Family Botanic Medicine.* The section on preparing medicines contained various botanical recipes, but with key ingredients left out. Agents filled in the blanks only after buyers pledged themselves to secrecy "under the penalty of forfeiting their word and honor, and all right to the use of the medicine."

During the 1820s and 1830s Thomsonian agents fanned out from New England through the southern and western United States urging self-reliant Americans to become their own physicians. Almost everywhere they met with success. By 1840 approximately one hundred thousand Family Rights had been sold, and Thomson estimated that about three million persons had adopted his system. In states as diverse as Ohio and Mississippi, perhaps as many as one-half the citizens were curing themselves the Thomsonian way.[5] And as Daniel Drake observed, the devotees of Thomsonianism were not "limited to the vulgar. Respectable and intelligent mechaniks, legislative and judicial officers, both state and federal barristers, ladies, ministers of the gospel, and even some of the medical profession 'who hold the eel of science by the tail' have become its converts and puffers."[6]

The Thomsonian rallying cry was "Every man his own physician."[7] Unlike many other sectarians, who simply wanted the public to exchange one kind of physician for another, the early Thomsonians seemed genuinely pleased with the prospect of a world without physicians. Given the Jacksonian temper of the times, their slogan had great popular appeal. It reflected both the widespread distrust of elites and the conviction that the head of an American family "should in medicine, as in religion and politics, think and act for himself."[8] It was high time, declared Thomson, for the common man to throw off the oppressive yoke of priests, lawyers, and physicians and assume his rightful place in a truly democratic society.[9]

On a more practical level, the Thomsonians argued persuasively that self-medication was safer than being "doctored to death."[10] Again they struck a responsive chord, for Americans in increasing numbers were growing suspicious of the purported benefits of repeated bleedings and calomel dosings. Common people were more likely to place their trust in the healing power of nature and the indigenous remedies that grew around them.[11] They could be sure that their domestically prepared medicines would be "pure, genuine, and unadulterated," unlike those often prepared by apothecaries, or worse yet, their apprentices.[12] Thomsonians frequently commented on the relative safety of their home treatments. "It has been generally remarked," wrote one, "that those families that employ no physicians, in cases of scarlet fever, canker rash, measles, and &c., lose a less number of children, than those who employ them."[13] Another could not recall "a single death from childhood disease" occurring under Thomsonian treatment.[14]

But Thomsonians offered more than safety. Being your own physician would not only save your life, promised one botanic manual, but your money as well.[15] After the initial outlay of twenty dollars, the Thomsonian family need never worry about exorbitant bills from physicians and apothecaries. This alone, thought one Thomsonian, would be sufficient inducement for most people to turn to domestic medicine.[16] The savings often were substantial; one New Hampshire family calculated theirs to be seventy-five dollars a year.[17]

Another unquestioned benefit of home treatment was convenience. "[T]he physician and the cure are always at hand," stressed another Thomsonian. "You have not to wander in the night to a distance, and the patient dying, to seek a doctor, with the agony pressing on your spirits, that your wife, or child, or friend may be dead on your return."[18] And where there were no physicians at all, domestic medicine was not only convenient but necessary. In the western states especially, which sometimes experienced shortages of physicians and apothecaries, self-treatment could be essential.[19] Here the Thomsonians were at a decided advantage, because, as Philip D. Jordan has noted, "most settlers had to supply themselves with drugs, and herbs were easier to secure than chemical mixtures and compounds."[20]

Finally, being your own physician allowed women to avoid the embarrassment of going to male physicians. By adopting Thomsonianism, wrote one advocate, women escaped "the necessity of consulting the other sex, with all its attendant indelicacy and mortification."[21] They also won the freedom to practice medicine in a limited way. Joseph Kett has recently argued that Thomsonianism, with its emphasis on the wife and mother as physician, opened medical practice to women "without forcing a confrontation of the sensitive question of whether a woman should ever treat a man other than her husband."[22]

With every person a physician, professional healers were left with few tasks indeed. Samuel Thomson, who opposed even Thomsonian infirmaries and medical schools, would have given them virtually none. If Thomsonian physicians were available, he argued, then people would no longer see the desirability of learning to treat themselves—and perhaps more important, though he did not mention it, they would no longer find it necessary to purchase his Family Rights.[23] Among orthodox Thomsonians, the sole function of physicians was educational. "The physician, instead of dealing out poison," explained one, "would deal out advice to his fellow men to live according to the dictates of nature."[24] He was not to be concerned about the prospect of losing his practice as home treatment increased. Instead, he was to expect to tire of his work after eight or ten years and "be happy to have the people take the burthen of the practice upon themselves."[25]

Not all Thomsonians, however, accepted such a restricted role for trained doctors. Some recommended resorting to physicians in cases of serious cuts, punctured arteries, broken bones, or unusual or dangerous diseases. This tolerance toward professionals became more common with the opening, over Thomson's adamant opposition, of botanic medical schools in the late 1830s. Naturally those associated with such institutions viewed domestic medicine in a different light from Thomson: home manuals were not to replace the physician but to supplement his efforts.[26] (This was also the opinion of Wooster Beach, founder of the rival Eclectic school of medicine and author of two works on home medicine.)[27] Acrimonious debates over such issues as medical education eventually rent the Thomsonians into hostile camps and precipitated the demise of the movement.

As Thomsonian strength began to wane in the 1840s, a new medical sect, homeopathy, was rising to national prominence.[28] Homeopathy was the invention of a regularly educated German physician, Samuel Hahnemann, who had grown dissatisfied with the heroics of orthodox practice. During the last decade of the eighteenth century, he began constructing an alternate system based in large part upon the healing power of nature and two fundamental principles, the law of similars and the law of infinitesimals. According to the first law, diseases are cured by medicines having the property of producing in healthy persons symptoms similar to those of the disease. An individual suffering from fever, for example, would be treated with a drug known to increase the pulse rate of a person in health. Hahnemann's second law held that medicines are more efficacious the smaller the dose, even as small as dilutions of up to one-millionth of a gram. Though regular practitioners—or allopaths as Hahnemann called them—ridiculed this theory, patients seldom suffered from homeopathic treatment and many flourished.

Following its appearance in this country in 1825, homeopathy rapidly grew into a major medical sect. By the outbreak of the Civil War there were nearly twenty-five hundred homeopathic physicians, concentrated largely in New England, New York, Pennsylvania, and the Midwest, and hundreds of thousands of devoted followers.[29] Homeopathy's appeal is not difficult to understand. Instead of the bleedings and purgings of the regulars, or the equally rigorous therapy of the Thomsonians, the homeopaths offered pleasant-tasting pills that produced no discomforting side effects. Such medication was particularly suitable for babies and small children. As the orthodox Oliver Wendell Holmes observed, homeopathy "does not offend the palate, and so spares the nursery those scenes of single combat in which infants were wont to yield at length to the pressure of the spoon and the imminence of asphyxia."[30] Perhaps because of its suitability for children, homeopathy won the support of large numbers of American women, who constituted approximately two-thirds of its patrons and who were among its most active propagators. "Many a woman, armed with her little stock of remedies, has converted an entire community," proudly reported the American Institute of Homeopathy.[31]

Central to the home practice of homeopathy was the "domestic kit," which consisted of a case of infinitesimal medicines and a guide. Scores if not hundreds of these were available during the nineteenth century in a variety of combinations ranging from small pocket cases with tiny guides to large family chests with thick volumes. Often the books appeared in foreign languages as well as English, and occasionally they included homeopathic treatments for domestic animals.[32]

The first such kit came from the hands of Constantine Hering, a Leipzig-educated physician who settled in Pennyslvania in the early 1830s and who did as much as any man to promote the cause of homeopathy in America. In 1835 he published the first part of *The Homeopathist, or Domestic Physician,* and three years later he completed the second part. These he sold, together with a small mahogany box of medicines, for five dollars (four dollars for the German edition). The box contained small numbered vials filled with "infinitesimal pills," the numbers on the vials corresponding to the numbered remedies in the book. Self-treatment, once a diagnosis was made, was thus reduced simply to taking a No. 8 or a No. 17 pill, or whatever the manual recommended.[33]

Since most homeopaths were, like Hahnemann and Hering, trained physicians, they understandably did not share the Thomsonian enthusiasm for making every man a physician. Besides, many were recent immigrants from Germany, uninfected by Jacksonian democracy. They envisioned only a limited role for domestic practice. Hering, for example, wrote his book not to replace the physician but to assist families in treating minor complaints and to provide medical advice for students, travelers, mariners, and "those living in remote parts of the country." Like virtually all his homeopathic colleagues, he urged his readers to seek qualified medical asssistance in serious cases.[34]

Several homeopathic domestic guides pointedly discouraged self-treatment. One warned that since even physicians could not safely treat themselves, ordinary persons should not think they could. George E. Shipman's popular *Homeopathic Family Guide* cautioned that "No *very* sensible person will ever attempt to treat himself or his family, who can obtain the advice of a well-qualified physician. If those fail too often, who make the study of disease and their remedies the sole business of their lives," wrote Shipman, "what success can they expect, who know little or nothing of either?"[35]

But regardless of their reservations about home treatment, homeopaths were well aware that the domestic kits were one of their most effective weapons in winning converts from the allopaths. The domestic guides, especially in the early days, were seen as "missionaries of truth" preparing the way for the arrival of homeopathic physicians. Thus most homeopaths viewed domestic manuals not as competitors, but "as necessary allies in the great work of reforming the medical state of the world."[36] Even allopaths did not dispute their effectiveness. Many an "impecunious practitioner" has failed to get a case, complained one regular, because of "Dr. Humphrey's book and box that preceded him in the domestic corner."[37]

The homeopaths also derived encouragment from the knowledge that their practice was relatively harmless—certainly safer than "the Old System of Physic," "whose gentlest weapons are lancets and cathartics." Even if the patient took the wrong medicine, there was no need for alarm, wrote Hering, "for Homeopathic medicine is so prepared that it will help, when it is the right one, but it will not injure should a mistake occur." The very worst possibility would be a slight delay in the healing process.[38] Readers of one manual were assured that "No life was ever lost by homeopathic medicine used carelessly, or otherwise," a point conceded by sarcastic allopaths. Homeopathy, wrote Dr. Holmes, "gives the ignorant, who have such an inveterate itch for dabbling in physic, a book and a doll's medicine chest, and lets them play doctors and doctoresses without fear of having to call in the coroner."[39]

Frederick Humphreys, further popularized homeopathy by simplifying home medication. A sometime professor in the Homeopathic Medical College of Pennsylvania, Humphreys broke with Hahnemann's rule of administering only one medicine at a time and instead recommended combinations of medicines for specific diseases, manufactured by his own Specific Homeopathic Medicine Company. Although some uncharitable colleagues called his invention "Homeopathic quackery," lay homeopaths seem to have thought otherwise. The sale of his two domestic guides, a large one to accompany his more expensive kits and a smaller one for his cheaper cases, was truly phenomenal. By the early 1890s, fifteen million copies of the latter work had appeared in five languages, twelve million of which had been distributed in the United States. In one year alone he printed three million copies.[40]

Despite the safety and popularity of these domestic kits and their acknowledged role in diffusing the principles of homeopathy, a few homeopaths questioned what they saw as an overemphasis on home medical care. John Ellis of Cleveland thought that books on preventive medicine were far more important "than any work on domestic medicine can possibly be," and claimed that his own *Family Homeopathy* was written primarily to direct attention to his earlier but often ignored work on *The Avoidable Causes of Disease*.[41] *The Family Journal of Homeopathy,* published by a group of St. Louis physicians, went even further in condemning "domestic practice of every description." "[W]e would prefer a good Allopath to prescribe for us than an ignorant or mongrel Homeopath," the editors declared.[42]

As the century progressed and homeopathy came to occupy a secure place in American medicine, homeopaths began directing their attention less to the general public and more toward their own profession.[43] The writing of Charles J. Hempel, who authored a *Homeopathic Domestic Physician* in 1846, reflects this change. After issuing two editions of his home guide, he became increasingly pessimistic about the value of domestic practice and decided, instead of preparing a third edition, to publish a volume on *Homeopathic Theory and Practice,* "designed both for the public and for students and practitioners."[44]

The domestic guides that continued to appear during the latter part of the century tended to be somewhat less comprehensive than their predecessors and to focus instead on emergency care and minor diseases. There is no longer any need to provide every person with the "knowledge of a physician," wrote one homeopath in 1887, "for the doctor himself is at hand in every village and hamlet of the land, ready at first summons to give advice and assistance far more valuable than that of any book."[45] This situation did not last long, however, if in fact it ever existed. Within a few decades homeopathy was fast fading from sight, and the question of homeopathic domestic practice had become moot.

To escape the most obvious pitfalls of allopathic practice, the Thomsonians had turned to botanic remedies and the homeopaths to their infinitesimal pills. A third sect, hydropathy, rejected drugs of every variety, whether botanic or mineral, in large or small doses. The hydropaths placed their trust solely in natural cures like fresh air, sunshine, exercise, proper (often vegetarian) diet, and, above all, water, which they used in every conceivable way.[46]

Hydropathy was a mélange of water treatments devised by a Silesian peasant, Vincent Priessnitz, to heal his wounds after accidentally being run over by a wagon. His therapy proved so successful that he opened his home in Graefenberg as a "water cure" and invited his ailing neighbors to submit their bodies to a bewildering variety of baths, packs, and wet bandages. When news of his methods reached the United States in the mid-1840s, it touched off a water-cure craze that continued unabated until the outbreak of the Civil War. Two regularly educated physicians, Joel Shew and Russell T. Trall, opened the first American water-cure establishments in New York City about 1843. A couple of years later, Mary Gove Nichols, an experienced woman health reformer, opened still a third water cure in the city. It was primarily these three pioneers—Shew, Trall, and Nichols—who introduced Americans to the new water system.

Among them they wrote perhaps a dozen volumes for domestic use. Throughout their writings run many of the themes commonly found in sectarian guides: the economy and absolute safety of their practice, the importance of prevention, and the advantages of self-reliance. On the question of making every man a physician, they fell somewhere between the early radical Thomsonians and the more moderate homeopaths. Since all three writers operated commercial water cures, they could hardly deny the value of professional care; yet they realized that relatively few people had access to such establishments or to hydropathic physicians, of which there were never many.[47]

In theory they saw little justification for limiting self-practice. The water treatments themselves were harmless, with the possible exception of the powerful douche, which one author warned should be used "with great caution, and always under the direction of an experienced hydropathic physician."[48] In Shew's opinion, hydropathy was "destined, not only to make the members of communities their own physicians for the most part, but to mitigate, in an unprecedented manner, the extent, the pains, and the perils of disease." The only time when professional assistance might be necessary was in the event of a serious injury, like a skull fracture.[49] Trall's attitude was basically the same. When the people become familiar with the principles of hydropathy and the laws of life and health, he predicted, "they will well-nigh emancipate themselves from all need of doctors of any sort." He thought home practitioners could successfully treat functional problems, which he estimated to be 99 percent of all ailments, but that they would probably need the skill of a trained surgeon for "mechanical injuries, displacements of parts, organic lesions, etc."[50]

Mrs. Nichols, the only nonphysician of the three, looked forward expectantly to the day when the spread of hydropathy would make physicians obsolete. Since a water-cure family seldom needed a physician more than once, she foresaw the end of medical practices outside the home. "Mothers learn to not only cure the disease of their families, but, what is more important,

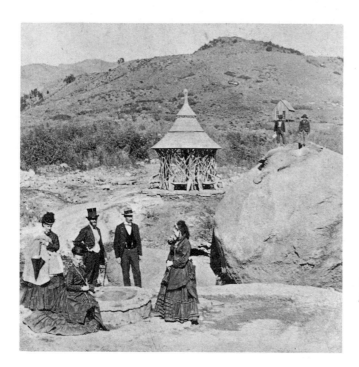

Visitors at Navajo Soda Springs Spa, Manitou Springs, Colorado (1872). Denver Public Library.

to keep them in health," she wrote in 1849. "The only way a Water Cure physician can live, is by constantly getting new patients, as the old ones are too thoroughly cured, and too well informed, to require further advice. This is a striking advantage to Water Cure patients, if not to Water Cure physicians."[51]

Like Thomsonians, hydropaths placed special emphasis on the role of women as providers and consumers of health care. In an age of few female doctors, roughly one-fifth of professional hydropaths were women.[52] Many water-curists of both sexes actively participated in the antebellum feminist movement, particularly as it related to freeing women from the dominance of male physicians. As part of their effort to effect the latter goal, they prepared domestic manuals instructing women on the care of their own bodies, as well as on the care of their families.[53]

One of the most successful means of popularizing all facets of hydropathy was the *Water-Cure Journal,* first published by Shew in 1845 and later edited by Trall. Beginning with the third volume, Shew promised to include considerable advice on domestic treatment, "thus enabling persons who cannot visit a hydropathic establishment, to prescribe for themselves." Those desiring more specific counsel than that printed in the journal were invited to correspond with the editor directly, on condition that they send a fee in advance.[54] Because of the scarcity of hydropathic physicians, several practitioners, including Mrs. Nichols, resorted to this semidomestic device.

Numerous letters from *Journal* readers demonstrate the great popularity of domestic hydropathy and the eagerness of home practitioners to relate their experiences. One elderly man from Missouri vividly described his treatment for fever in the following letter to the publishers:

. . . I put the patient in a hogshead that I keep for bathing. I have him go entirely under water, head and all, for three or four times, keeping his head under each time as long as he can conveniently hold his breath; then let him dabble in it up to the chin until the heat is reduced to the normal temperature, and the patient feels comfortable. . . . When I have no convenience for bathing, and, in fact, sometimes, as a matter of preference, I pour water on the patient's head, instead of bathing; and, surprising as it may seem, this always has the same effect that bathing has. . . . I have the patient lie with the head over the edge or side of the bed, so that the water will not wet the bedding. I then get a bucket of the coldest water. . . . The cure is completed in a few minutes, and it is a permanent cure, and a cure that all persons can perform at home without any inconvenience.[55]

John Harvey Kellogg (of cornflake fame), became the most prolific writer on domestic hydropathy—or hydrotherapy, as it came to be called—during the late nineteenth and early twentieth centuries, authoring such works as *The Household Manual of Domestic Hygiene, Ladies' Guide in Health and Disease, The Household Monitor of Health,* and *The Home Hand-Book of Domestic Hygiene and Rational Medicine,* which sold nearly a hundred thousand copies during its first twenty-five years.[56] Kellogg was the last of the major writers of domestic hydropathic guides, but well into the twentieth century there appeared an occasional home manual advocating hydrotherapy as the safest of all therapies.[57] These books, however, were largely devoid of sectarian spirit and probably differed more from Shew's and Trall's early handbooks than from the orthodox guides of the day.

The brief look at sectarian domestic medicine reveals something of the extent to which home health care permeated American society during the nineteenth century. For literally millions of Americans, the sectarian domestic guides served as primary care physicians. While it is true that much of the sectarian literature simply reflected orthodox concerns with cost, convenience, and accessibility of doctors, in many respects the sectarian tradition was unique: in its exploitation of the therapeutic weaknesses of regular medicine, in its more ready acceptance of domestic medicine as a substitute for professional health care, and in its missionary zeal. In view of the effectiveness of domestic medicine in making and holding sectarian converts, it is no exaggeration to say that home health care was the foundation upon which the American medical sects were built.

NOTES

I wish to thank Blanche L. Singer, of the Middleton Medical Library, University of Wisconsin, and Janet Schulze Numbers for their assistance in the preparation of this paper.

1. See Alex Berman, "The Impact of the Nineteenth-Century Botanico Medical Movement on American Pharmacy and Medicine" (Ph.D. diss., University of Wisconsin, 1954), 92–93.
2. John Gunn, *Gunn's Domestic Medicine, or Poor Man's Friend,* 1st rev.ed. (Philadelphia: G. V. Raymond, 1839). On the popularity of Gunn's book, see Madge E. Pickard and R. Carlyle Buley, *The Midwest Pioneer: His Ills, Cures, and Doctors* (New York: Henry Schuman, 1946), 93.

3. Berman's unpublished dissertation remains the most thorough treatment of Thomsonianism"; but see also Alex Berman, "The Thomsonian Movement and Its Relation to American Pharmacy and Medicine," *Bulletin of the History of Medicine* 25 (1951): 405–428; 519–538; Pickard and Buley, *The Midwest Pioneer*, 167–198; Joseph F. Kett, *The Formation of the American Medical Profession: The Role of Institutions, 1780–1860* (New Haven, CT: Yale University Press, 1968), 97–131; and James Harvey Young, *The Toadstool Millionaires: A Social History of Patent Medicines in America before Federal Regulation* (Princeton, NJ: Princeton University Press, 1961), 44–57.

4. Samuel Thomson, *New Guide to Health: or, Botanic Family Physician,* 2nd ed. (Boston: For the author, 1825), 1: 42–45.

5. Berman, "Nineteenth-Century Botanico Medical Movement," 150–52.

6. Daniel Drake, "The People's Doctors," *Western Journal of Medical & Physical Sciences* 407, (1829), quoted ibid., 42–43.

7. See Thomson, *New Guide to Health,* 1: 10. This motto, or variations of it, appears in numerous botanic works on domestic medicine.

8. William Procter, Jr., *American Journal of Pharmacy* 26: (1854), 570; quoted in Berman, "Nineteenth-Century Botanico Medical Movement," 40–41.

9. Thomson, *New Guide to Health,* 2: 5.

10. Horton Howard, *Howard's Domestic Medicine,* new enl. ed. (Philadelphia: Duane Rulison, 1866).

11. See, for example, Elisha Smith, *The Botanic Physician; Being a Compendium of the Practice of Physic, upon Botanical Principles* (New York: Murphy and Bingham, 1830), vi.

12. L. Sperry, *The Botanic Family Physician, or The Secret of Curing Diseases with Vegetable Proportions* (Cornwall, VT: By the author, 1843), 5.

13. Benjamin Colby, *A Guide to Health: Being an Exposition of the Principles of the Thomsonian System of Practice* (Nashua, NH: Charles T. Gill, 1844), x.

14. J. W. Comfort, *Thomsonian Practice of Midwifery* (Philadelphia: Aaron Comfort, 1845), iii.

15. F. K. Robertson and Silas Wilcox, *The Book of Health, or Thomsonian Theory and Practice of Medicine* (Bennington, VT: J. I. C. & A. S. C. Cook, 1843), 5.

16. Howard, *Howard's Domestic Medicine,* 427.

17. Colby, *A Guide to Health,* x.

18. Simon Abbott, *The Southern Botanic Physician* (Charleston: For the author, 1844), ix.

19. P. E. Sanborn urged husbands emigrating west to learn the art of midwifery, since "many females suffer and die in some parts of the West, for want of medical skill and attention." Sanborn, *The Sick Man's Friend* (Taunton, MA: By the author, 1835), 237.

20. Philip D. Jordan, "The Eclectic of St. Clairsville," *Ohio State Archaeological & Historical Quarterly* 56 (October 1947): 391.

21. Howard, *Howard's Domestic Medicine,* 286.

22. Kett, *The Formation of the American Medical Profession,* 119.

23. Samuel Thomson, Editorial, *Thomsonian Manual* 1 (Aug. 15,1836): 153.

24. Colby, *A Guide to Health,* viii.

25. Robertson and Wilcox, *The Book of Health,* p. 19.

26. See, for example, Wm. H. Cook. *Woman's Hand-Book of Health: A Guide for the Wife, Mother and Nurse,* 5th ed. (Cincinnati, OH: Wm. H. Cook, 1871). Cook was Professor of Botany, Therapeutics, and Materia Medica in the Physio-Medical Institute.

27. Wooster Beach, *The American Practice Condensed, or the Family Physician,* 10th ed. (New York: James McAlister, 1847), xv. Beach also published *The Family*

Physician; or The Reformed System of Medicine on Vegetable or Botanical Principles (New York: By the author, 1842).

28. On homeopathy in America, see Martin Kaufman, *Homeopathy in America: The Rise and Fall of a Medical Heresy* (Baltimore, MD: John Hopkins University Press, 1971); Harris L. Coulter, *Divided Legacy: A History of the Schism in Medical Thought* (Washington, D.C.: McGrath Publishing Co., 1973) III; and Kett, *The Formation of the American Medical Profession*, 132–164.

29. Coulter, *Divided Legacy* III: 101–110.

30. Oliver Wendell Holmes, "Some More Recent Views on Homeopathy," *Atlantic Monthly* 187 (December 1857), quoted ibid., 114.

31. Ibid., 114–16.

32. See, for example, C. S. and George E. Halsey, *Halsey's Homeopathic Guide: For Families, Travelers, Missionaries, Pioneers, Miners, Farmers, Stock Raisers, Horse Owners, Dog Fanciers, Poultry Keepers* (Chicago: C. S. and George E. Halsey, 1885). Domestic manuals appear with great frequency in Thomas Lindsley Bradford, *Homeopathic Bibliography of the United States, from the Year 1825 to the Year 1891, Inclusive* (Philadelphia: Boericke and Tafel, 1892).

33. C. Hering, *The Homeopathist, or Domestic Physician*, 2 parts (Philadelphia: J. G. Wesselhoeft, 1835, 1838); Coulter, *Divided Legacy* III: 101–2; Bradford, *Homeopathic Bibliography*, 145.

34. Hering, *The Homeopathist*, 1: 2–3; ibid. 2: 241.

35. Morton M. Eaton, *Eaton's Domestic Practice for Parents and Nurses* (Cincinnati, OH: M. M. Eaton, Jr., and Co., 1882), 77; George E. Shipman, *The Homeopathic Family Guide*, 2nd ed. (Chicago: C. S. Halsey, 1865), ix.

36. J. H. Pulte, *Homeopathic Domestic Physician; Containing the Treatment of Diseases, with Popular Explanations on Anatomy, Physiology, Hygiene, and Hydropathy* (Cincinnati: H. W. Derby and Co., 1850), iv–v. See also E. H. Ruddock, *The Stepping Stone to Homeopathy and Health*, ed. Wm. Boericke, new Am. ed. (Philadelphia: Hahnemann Publishing House, 1890), 10.

37. Quoted in Coulter, *Divided Legacy* III: 117.

38. Egbert Guernsey, *The Gentleman's Hand-Book of Homeopathy; Especially for Travelers, and for Domestic Practice* (Boston: Otis Clapp, 1855), iv; Hering, *The Homeopathist* 1: 7; John Epps, *Domestic Homeopathy*, ed. George W. Cook, 4th Am. ed. (Boston: Otis Clapp, 1849), 8.

39. E. R. Ellis, *Homeopathic Family Guide and Information for the People*, 2nd ed. (Detroit: By the author, 1882), ii; Holmes, "Some More Recent Views on Homeopathy," 187, quoted in Coulter, *Divided Legacy* III: 116.

40. Frederick Humphreys, *Manual of Specific Homeopathy* (New York: Humphrey's Specific Homeopathic Medicine Company, 1869); *Humphrey's Homeopathic Mentor or Family Adviser* (New York: Humphrey's Specific Homeopathic Medicine Company, 1876); Bradford, *Homeopathic Bibliography*, 167. The reference to "Homeopathic quackery" is from J. S. Douglas, *Practical Homeopathy for the People*, 15th ed. (Milwaukee, MN: Lewis Sherman, 1894), iii.

41. John Ellis, *Personal Experience of a Physician* (Philadelphia: Hahnemann Publishing House, 1892), 85–87.

42. "Domestic Practice—No. 2," *Family Journal of Homeopathy* 1 (July 1854): 105. See also Guernsey's reply to the criticisms against domestic practice: Guernsey, *The Gentleman's Hand-Book of Homeopathy*, iv.

43. "Progress of Homeopathy," *Homeopathic Sun* 1 (September 1868): 12.

44. Charles J. Hempel, *The Homeopathic Domestic Physician* (New York: Wm. Radde, 1868), iii.

45. Henry G. Hanchett, *The Elements of Modern Domestic Medicine* (New York: Charles T. Hurlburt, 1887), 3.

46. On hydropathy in America, see Harry B. Weiss and Howard R. Kemble, *The Great American Water-Cure Craze: A History of Hydropathy in the United States* (Trenton, NJ: Past Times Press, 1967); and Marshall Scott Legan, "Hydropathy in America; a Nineteenth Century Panacea," *Bulletin of the History of Medicine* 45 (1971): 267–80.

47. Weiss and Kemble, *The Great American Water-Cure Craze* (44), were able to identify only 241 American hydropathic physicians.

48. David A. Harsha, *The Principles of Hydropathy, or the Invalid's Guide to Health and Happiness* (Albany, NY: E. H. Pease & Co., 1852), 41.

49. Jocl Shew, *The Hydropathic Family Physician* (New York: Fowler and Wells, 1854), iii; Shew, *The Water-Cure Manual: A Popular Work* (New York: Fowler and Wells, 1855), 132. Shew's *Hand-Book of Hydropathy* (New York: Wiley and Putnam, 1844) was probably the first American domestic guide to hydropathy.

50. R. T. Trall, American preface to William Horsell, *Hydropathy for the People* (New York: Fowler and Wells, 1855), iii; Trall, *The Hydropathic Encyclopedia: A System of Hydropathy and Hygiene* (New York: Fowler and Wells, 1851) I: 295.

51. Mary S. Gove Nichols, *Experience in Water-Cure: A Familiar Exposition of the Principles and Results of Water Treatment, in the Cure of Acute and Chronic Diseases* (New York: Fowler & Wells, 1852), 10.

52. Weiss and Kemble, *The Great American Water-Cure Craze,* 44.

53. See, for example, Mary S. Gove, *Lectures to Women on Anatomy and Physiology, with an Appendix on Water Cure* (New York: Harper and Brothers, 1846); and M. Augusta Fairchild, *How to Be Well, or Common-Sense Medical Hygiene* (New York: Fowler & Wells, 1880).

54. *Water-Cure Journal* 2 (Nov. 1, 1846): 168; ibid. 6 (1848): 138. An example of how domestic practice supplemented the use of water-cure establishments is found in the diary of Mrs. Angeline Stevens Andrews, 1863–1864 (C. Burton Clark Collection, Heritage Room, Loma Linda University Library).

55. Abraham Millar to Fowler and Wells, Nov. 30, 1850, quoted in Trall, *Hydropathic Encyclopedia* II: 81–82.

56. (John Harvey Kellogg), *The Household Manual of Domestic Hygiene, Foods and Drinks, Common Diseases, Accidents and Emergencies, and Useful Hints and Recipes* (Battle Creek, MI: Modern Medicine Publishing Co., 1893); Kellogg, *Ladies' Guide in Health and Disease* (Battle Creek, MI: Modern Medicine Publishing Co., 1893); Kellogg, *The Household Monitor of Health* (Battle Creek, MI: Good Health Publishing Co., 1891); Kellogg, *The Home Hand-Book of Domestic Hygiene and Rational Medicine,* rev. ed. (Battle Creek, MI: Modern Medicine Publishing Co., 1906); the last work was first published in 1880. Kellogg's older half-brother Merritt also wrote domestic manuals; see (M. G. Kellogg), *The Hygienic Family Physician: A Complete Guide for the Preservation of Health, and the Treatment of the Sick without Medicine* (Battle Creek, MI: Health Reformer, 1874); and M. G. Kellogg, *The Bath: Its Use and Application* (Battle Creek, MI: Health Reformer, 1873).

57. See, for example, Newton Evans, Percy T. Magan, and George Thomason, eds., *The Home Physician and Guide to Health* (Mountain View, CA: Pacific Press, 1923), and Hubert O. Swartout, *Guide to Health* (Mountain View, CA: Pacific Press, 1938).

Part Two

THE LEAVEN OF TENDER HUMANITY

Women Enter the Medical Profession

Introduction

IF some male physicians thought women would be an ennobling force in nineteenth-century medicine, many women were certain of it. Vowing to bring the "leaven of tender humanity that women represent" to the profession, thousands of nineteenth-century women overcame enormous opposition and obtained medical training. By the century's end, over seven thousand women were serving as physicians. Their numbers included not only white Protestants, but also blacks (over one hundred), Jews, and members of new immigrant groups.

Of course, the path to this professional success had not been easy. Older practitioners, participants in the early battles, urged their young colleagues to remember and respect the mid-century pioneers. It could be fairly said that every nineteenth-century woman doctor was a pioneer. At the same time, some stood out so clearly that no discussion of the emergence of the American woman physician could fail to focus upon them.

In New York, doctors Emily and Elizabeth Blackwell founded the first hospital in the world run entirely by women. In Boston, Dr. Harriot Hunt's application to Harvard Medical School signaled the beginning of the campaign for women's entry into the established medical schools. In the same city, Dr. Marie Zakrzewska founded the New England Hospital for Women and Children, which early advocated some of the best European scientific practices. In Philadelphia, Dr. Ann Preston served as Dean and guiding light of the Woman's Medical College of Pennsylvania, the first regular medical college for women in the world. In all these cities, Dr. Mary Putnam Jacobi worked to upgrade the medical education and training of women physicians, and by her own brilliant example, paved the way into the male medical establishment.

Together, aided by "generous men and noble women" across the nation, these six pathbreakers built a woman's medical sphere that supported hundreds of Victorian women in their bids for medical education. As the turn of the century approached, their main goal of full integration seemed so close that this separate sphere, always seen as a temporary expedience, was abandoned.

In her later years, Marie Zakrzewska wondered whether there would ever be a monument to the early pioneers. Happily, there are many. Hospitals throughout the United States bear their names and enshrine their memories. Medical outreach programs such as the Visiting Nurse Service, a product of the nineteenth-century woman physician's commitment to social welfare, still serve the needy today. And the growing demand for a more humanistic approach to medical care is a direct legacy from the nineteenth-century women's medical movement. Perhaps it is the inspiring story of victory over social mistrust and self-doubt that these women left behind that will be the most enduring "monument" of all.

The Female Student Has Arrived

The Rise of the Women's Medical Movement

REGINA MORANTZ-SANCHEZ

WHEN the young audience attending the fall session of Geneva Medical College in upstate New York listened to the dean of the faculty one morning in 1847, they probably only dimly comprehended the historical significance of the gentleman's words. In quavering tones, he spoke to them of a letter from a prominent physician in Philadelphia and sought their response to the writer's unconventional request.

For several months this physician had been preceptor of a lady student who had already attended a course of lectures in Cincinnati. He wished her to have the opportunity to graduate from an eastern medical college, but his efforts in securing her acceptance had thus far ended in failure. A country college like Geneva, he hoped, would prove more open-minded. If not, the young woman's only recourse would be to seek training in Europe. As the

Reprinted, with changes, from Regina Morantz-Sanchez's "From Art to Science: Women Physicians in American Medicine, 1600–1980," the introduction to *In Her Own Words: Oral Histories of Women in Medicine,* eds. Regina Morantez-Sanchez, Cynthia Stodola Pomerleau, and Carol Hansen Fenichel (Westport, CT: Greenwood Press, 1982). Used by permission of the author.

dean spoke, a silence fell upon the room. For several moments the students sat transfixed as he concluded his remarks with the comment that the faculty would accede to the request only if the students favored acceptance unanimously.

The students themselves did not realize that the faculty was emphatically opposed to the admission of a woman. Not wanting to assume the sole responsibility for denying the request, the faculty had thought that the students would reject the proposal, and they planned to use the action of a united student body to justify their own response.

Stephen Smith, then a bright young member of the class and later a prominent New York physician and public-health advocate, witnessed the ensuing events. Over half a century later, at a memorial service for his longtime friend and colleague, Elizabeth Blackwell, he recalled the following:

> But the Faculty did not understand the tone and temper of the class. For a minute or two, after the departure of the Dean, there was a pause, then the ludicrousness of the situation seemed to seize the entire class, and a perfect Babel of talk, laughter, and cat-calls followed. Congratulations upon the new source of excitement were everywhere heard, and a demand was made for a class meeting to take action on the faculty's communication. . . . At length the question was put to vote, and the whole class arose and voted "Aye" with waving of handkerchiefs, throwing up of hats, and all manner of vocal demonstrations.
>
> A fortnight or more had passed, and the incident . . . had ceased to interest anyone, when one morning the Dean came into the class-room, evidently in a state of unusual agitation. The class took alarm, fearing some great calamity was about to befall the College, possibly its closure under the decree of the court that it was a public nuisance. He stated, with trembling voice, that . . . the female student . . . had arrived.
>
> With this introduction . . . a lady . . . entered, whom he formally introduced as Miss Elizabeth Blackwell. . . . A hush fell upon the class as if each member had been stricken with paralysis. A death-like stillness prevailed during the lecture, and only the newly arrived student took notes. She retired with the Professor, and thereafter came in with him and sat on the platform during the lecture.[1]

Although this anecdote perhaps suggested that the formal movement to train women in medicine began somewhat inauspiciously, the truth of the matter is that the "social groundwork" for women entering the medical profession had already been laid by the time Elizabeth Blackwell applied to Geneva. Of course, these pioneer women had a difficult time of it in the beginning; nevertheless, a number of factors came together in the mid-nineteenth century to make their entrance into the profession possible, though it had not been only fifty years before. First, there were the structural growing pains of a profession in transition. The advances in medical science had begun to call traditional heroic therapeutics into question. Meanwhile, the discovery of anaesthesia at the end of the 1840s challenged older concepts of professionalism in a different way. Before anaesthesia, the necessity of inflicting pain on patients constituted an integral part of the self-image and ideology of physicians.[2] Empathy was to be balanced with cool detachment—and the best physician knew that his role was to cure, not to soothe. The necessity for manly detachment—which women, it was argued, could not achieve—was

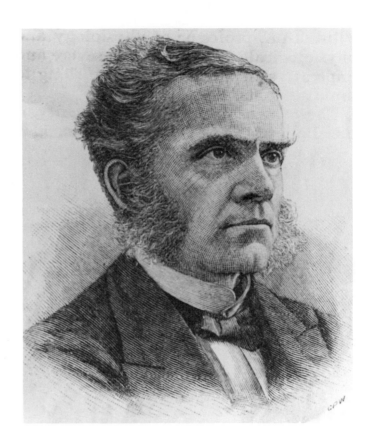

Dr. Stephen Smith, 1823–1922 (1860s). New York Academy of Medicine.

often used as an objection to women in medicine. But the use of ether and chloroform weakened this argument and "feminized" medicine by undermining more generally the heroic image of the physician.[3]

Coupled with changes in medical science and technology were institutional growing pains. Efforts to raise the standards of medical education floundered, while proprietary medical schools proliferated. Jacksonian anti-elitism added to the profession's worries, as did the appearance of a lay health reform movement, often connected in spirit to the rise of medical sectarianism. In addition, sectarians and health reformers often welcomed women into their schools and societies. Since sectarians established their own professional institutions, the abandonment of licensing legislation and the ease of access to a medical degree actually served in this period to maintain a professional identity for all medical practitioners by conferring the title of doctor on a large proportion of them. This temporary fluidity allowed women who wished to achieve professional status to do so before definitions of professionalism crystallized once more.[4]

These were the conditions that made the medical profession vulnerable to the entrance of women. But there were also changes taking place in the social definition of woman's role in the nineteenth century that made more and more middle-class women comfortable with the idea of studying medicine.

The onset of industrialization brought about important alterations in the organization of work and family life. The separation of home and work reduced the father's role in domestic life while the mother and children found themselves alone in the household. Accompanying these social and economic changes was an elaborate ideology based on the idea of separate spheres for men and women. The world of men was considered "public," the world of women "private." Of course, this new ideology of domesticity, on the surface at least, merely reaffirmed woman's traditional connection with the private sphere. In theory, there was really nothing terribly new about a limited and sex-specific role for women in the home. But in reality, the ideology of domesticity contained within it kernels of radical change. As many recent historians have not hesitated to point out, it gave women extraordinary new power in the private sphere. The ideology of domesticity romanticized both the family and woman's role within it. As Americans were forced increasingly to cope with the problems of industrialization in the nineteenth century, the family became for them a kind of ideological touchstone for all that was good, beautiful, and true. Gradually women, now defined as the moral and spiritual center of that family, were given a central role in the preservation of values that were intended to inform the institutions of society at large. Woman's role was suddenly invested with cosmic moral significance. When emphasis was placed on the socially transforming aspects of woman's role in the home, the results proved revolutionary. Middle-class women could and very soon, as we shall see, did use their newly gained power over domestic life to establish a base for self-assertion in the public sphere. Making the home a model for social interaction, they played an unprecedented part in what became the reformist critique of industrializing America. While the ideology of domesticity could be used by social conservatives to keep women in the home, in reality it was used just as powerfully by feminists to push for the widest possible definition of woman's sphere. Many middle-class women who took their moral and social role seriously understood from the very beginning that to purify society, some women might indeed have to enter it.[5] Elizabeth Blackwell was one of these women, as were most of the early generations of women physicians.

Women doctors, then, belong to that group among nineteenth-century women that historians have labeled "domestic feminists."[6] They viewed their campaign to study and practice medicine as part of a larger effort to adapt traditional concepts of womanhood to the demands of an unstable, complex, and rapidly industrializing society. This redefinition explicitly called for a more intensive role within the family for all women and implicitly demanded a more comprehensive role for at least some women in society at large. Rarely did this early generation of women physicians challenge the cult of domesticity. Indeed, they were genuinely comfortable with the concept of separate sexual spheres, because it allowed them to argue that women, by virtue of their special skills at nurturance, had a role in medicine that could compensate for and be complementary to the role and achievements of men.[7] Elizabeth and Emily Blackwell called women physicians the "connecting link" between the science of the medical profession and the everyday life of women, arguing that women physicians were "for the purpose of occupying positions which men cannot fully occupy, and exercising an influence which men cannot wield at all."[8] For many women physicians, this meant a special concern for the family and for preventive medicine. They believed that men had sorely neglected prevention, and thus they adopted it as their special province. "We should give to man cheerfully the curative department, and women the preventative," announced Dr. Harriot Hunt in 1852, stating further, "The female physician must be preventative. She must look upon life through sanitary channels." So too agreed Dr. Amanda C. Price, who asked in her 1871 senior thesis at the Woman's Medical College of Pennsylvania, "How many men do we find teaching the laws of health . . . ? It seems to be their ambition to cure disease, and very seldom do any of them think it worth their while to teach their patients how to prevent a return of their maladies." Price's classmate Prudence Saur agreed. Being a physician meant more than being able to "diagnose and treat Scarlatina." "How much more God-like," she observed, "to *prevent* as well as *cure!*"[9]

Armed with the conviction that medical science needed the "leaven of tender humanity that women represent," hundreds of women sought medical training in the decades following Elizabeth Blackwell's graduation from Geneva Medical College.[10] By 1880, a handful of medical schools accepted women on a regular basis, but still dissatisfied with the progress of medical coeducation, female pioneers founded five "regular" and several sectarian women's medical colleges. They built dispensaries and hospitals to provide clinical training for female graduates. By the end of the nineteenth century, female physicians numbered between 4 and 5 percent of the profession, a figure that remained relatively stable until the 1960s.[11]

The majority of male medical professionals did not welcome their female colleagues, whom they viewed as an economic threat in a profession already burdened with an oversupply of practitioners. When the graduates of the orthodox female medical colleges sought admission to local and national medical societies, they were rejected on grounds that their training was either irregular or of poor quality. Opponents held women's allegedly inferior training against them, yet denied them access to the type of education that was acceptable and often refused to consult with them or ostracized those male practitioners who did. These insults were perpetrated despite the fact that a fair number of medical women received excellent training in the nineteenth century. A comparative study of curricular and clinical offerings in several nineteenth-century medical schools suggests that those women who earned their diplomas at the orthodox women's colleges endured a vigorous, demanding, and refreshingly progressive course of study. Other women, self-conscious about their inadequacies and determined to procure proper preparation, sought postgraduate training in Europe.[12]

The regular medical profession objected on many levels to the entrance of women into its ranks. In the first place, the vast majority of doctors were traditionalists who subscribed to the cult of domesticity with the same intense tenacity as their nonmedical brethren. Placing women on a pedestal and cementing them firmly within the confines of the home, they worried that women who sought professional training would avoid the responsibility to raise children and thus disrupt American family life. Believers in the cult of domesticity felt that because women kept men respectable through the "home influence," their venturing out into the world could demoralize both sexes. Woman's mission was not to pursue science but "to rear the offspring and even fan the flame of piety, patriotism and love upon the sacred altar of her home."[13]

Other physicians cited woman's inferior intellect, her passivity of mind, her physical weakness, and her tendency toward hysteria. John Ware's conviction that medical education, with its "ghastly" rituals and "blood and agony" in the dissecting room, would harden women's hearts and leave them bereft of softness and empathy reappeared in elaborate guise. The *Boston Medical and Surgical Journal* continued to grumble about increasing economic competition.[14] More subtle and more insidious was the fear that an influx of women would alter the image of the profession by feminizing it in unacceptable ways. "The primary requisite for a good surgeon," insisted Edmund Andrews, "is *to be a man,*—a man of courage. . . ." Few physicians were prepared to surrender their masculinity gracefully. One Boston doctor taunted women physicians with the remark, "If they cannot stride a mustang or mend bullet holes, so much the better for an enterprizing and skillful practitioner of the sterner sex."[15]

Opponents of women physicians were neither scientific nor consistent. They praised women's abilities as nurses but rejected their competence in medicine; they offered their arguments for female inferiority, vulnerability, and dependence alongside their claims for women's moral superiority and domestic responsibility. There were even some medical men who successfully hid their prejudices under the cloak of science. In the 1870s and the 1880s, these physicians managed to transfer the grounds for the argument over female nature from the spiritual to the somatic.

Rallying around a book entitled *Sex in Education: A Fair Chance for Girls,* published in 1873, by E. H. Clarke, a Harvard professor, they based their case against women almost entirely on biological factors. Menstruation was depicted as mysteriously debilitating and higher education in any subject as sapping the energy needed for the normal development of the reproductive organs. The results, lamented Clarke with total seriousness, were "those grievous maladies which torture a woman's earthly existence: leuchorrhoea [sic], amenorrhea, dysmenorrhea, chronic and acute ovaritis, proplapsus uteri, hysteria, neuralgia, and the like."[16] He concluded that higher education for women produced "monstrous brains and puny bodies; abnormally active cerebration and abnormally weak digestion; flowing thought and constipated bowels."[17]

The biological argument proved particularly vexing to feminists. M. Carey Thomas, the indomitable president of Bryn Mawr and a fierce supporter of women physicians, recalled years later, "We did not know when we began whether women's health could stand the strain of education. We were haunted in those days, by the clanging chains of that gloomy little specter, Dr. Edward H. Clarke's *Sex in Education.*"[18]

When the feminist community launched a full-scale counterattack against the Clarke thesis, women physicians armed themselves with original research and statistics to lend scientific respectability to the campaign. Mary Putman

Jacobi, for example, won Harvard Medical School's esteemed Boylston Prize in 1876 for her essay "The Question of Rest for Women During Menstruation." Her study challenged conservative medical opinion with sophisticated statistical analyses and case studies. In 1881, Emily and Augusta Pope, graduates of the New England Female Medical College, and Emma Call, an early alumna of the University of Michigan Medical School, published a survey of women physicians sponsored by the American Social Science Association. While serving as staff physicians at the New England Hospital for Woman and Children, they summarized the results of their findings on the health of 430 women doctors and concluded that "some unnecessary anxiety has been wasted on this point." They went on to say, "We do not think it would be easy to find a better record of health among an equal number of women, taken at random, from all over the country."[19] Women physicians who held resident positions at the various women's colleges painstakingly monitored the physiological effects of higher education on their charges. Several of these women published studies that added to the growing body of scientific literature that seriously questioned Clarke's thesis. Indeed, one of the important contributions woman physicians made to the feminist movement in the late nineteenth century arose from their willingness to challenge on scientific and empirical grounds the somatic definition of woman's nature and to push toward innovative and less biologically constricting approaches to female health and hygiene.[20]

Women physicians also made important contributions to feminism by their example. Medicine attracted larger numbers of women in the nineteenth century than any of the other so-called learned professions. Feminists concerned with women's professional advancement particularly wanted women to have equal access to medical training. M. Carey Thomas gave the women physician a central role in the "furtherance of the intellectual life of women in general." So too did Mary Putnam Jacobi, who argued that there would "be no really higher education for women, until at least one profession is open to them for which such education is indispensable, and medicine is most definitely available for this purpose." The fellowship of common membership in a profession, Jacobi believed, afforded a model to women in other occupations. As women carved a place for themselves in medicine, "whose tests are more strict, whose rewards are more precise, and whose practical bearing is more powerful [the position of women in] literature, education, art and science will be better defined and valued," she postulated.[21]

Physicians like Jacobi, who won the grudging respect of male colleagues, provided strong, vigorous role models for younger women wishing to enter the professions at the end of the nineteenth century.[22] Women doctors who married (and between one-fifth and one-third did) furnished a feminist alternative to the constrictions of traditional Victorian family relationships. Nineteenth-century feminist theory devoted much attention to the restructuring of male-female relationships within marriage, but women physicians confronted the issue in personal terms.[23] "A woman can love and respect her family just as much if not more," asserted Dr. Georgiana Glenn, a wife and mother herself, "when she feels that she is supporting herself and adding to their comfort and happiness." Mary Putnam Jacobi, married and the mother of two children, frankly conceded that matrimony complicated professional life, but she also believed that raising children increased vigor and vitality in healthy women and "a good deal more than compensates for the difficulties involved in caring for them."[24]

Professionally as well as personally, women doctors viewed themselves as having a special relationship to motherhood and family life. "A woman Doctor," wrote Dr. Eliza Mosher to her sister in 1887, "holds a position of greater responsibility than does a man. So many questions come to her which are never asked of men . . . and her relation to families and family life is a very intimate and sacred one." In their approach to treatment, most nineteenth-century women physicians took their role as teachers of hygiene with great seriousness. "Women physicians," wrote Frances A. Rutherford in 1893, "were early selected as teachers of hygiene, were friends of women teachers, helped them and mothers to see the necessity of the development of the children in a threefold manner, mentally, morally and physically." Besides lecturing at mothers' meetings, women's temperance organizations, social purity groups, and women's clubs, woman doctors taught hygiene in the newly established women's colleges and published books and pamphlets on family hygiene and female health.[25]

The available evidence suggests that their hospitals and dispensaries gave scrupulous attention to the physician's heuristic role and anticipated the hospital social service departments of the twentieth century. The New York Infirmary, for example, was one of the first hospitals founded by women to establish the position of "sanitary visitor." The post usually was filled by a young graduate of the medical school who wished to gain further clinical experience. The intern was expected to go into the slums not only to treat emergency cases but also to teach cleanliness, proper ventilation, nutrition, and family hygiene. Other women's hospitals followed suit. In the Woman's Hospital in Cleveland, Ohio, interns did not confine their work "entirely to curing the sick." Here, as in New York, employment was found for those patients who needed it, and instruction was offered "in the laws of health" and in "the care and diet of children." Hospitals run by women physicians in Chicago, San Francisco, and Boston recorded similar goals.[26]

Individuals in private practice also felt it was their duty to enlighten as well as to heal. Evelyn Garrigue, a New York physician and an admirer of Elizabeth Blackwell's reform ideas, wrote to her in 1899 that she had distributed copies of Blackwell's pamphlet, *Counsel to Parents on the Moral Education of the Young,* to her patients, and that she now had a volume circulating "among some very noble tenement house patients, slaving themselves to protect their children from the evils to which they are exposed." Garrigue felt particularly grateful to Blackwell because the older woman's pamphlets represented a "powerful aid in my work." She added, "Since coming into medicine and getting my eyes opened to evils . . . I have been stirred to the innermost depth of my being . . . and when your sister kindly lent me your 'Essays in Medical Sociology' . . . I was able to gain a clear exposition of them with reference to the duty of the physician." It hardly seems necessary to add that it was a woman's medical college, the New York Infirmary, that became the first institution in the country to establish a faculty chair in preventative medicine, in 1868.[27]

Nineteenth-century medical women successfully managed to secure a place in medicine by creating a professional role that was believed to bridge the gap between the public and private. Their role applied "domestic" values to larger communal concerns and utilized the scientific and technical advances made in the public realm for the improvement of life at home. In justifying their extradomestic activity by using the Victorian stereotype of "woman as mother," female medical educators and their supporters differed little from female moral reformers and other nineteenth-century social feminists who professed a home-based ideology in order to introduce significant numbers of women to activity in the public sphere.

NOTES

1. Stephen Smith, M.D., "A Woman Student in a Medical College," *In Memory of Dr. Elizabeth Blackwell and Dr. Emily Blackwell* (New York: Academy of Medicine, 1911), 3–19

2. Martin Pernick, "Medical Profession: I: Medical Professionalism," in *Encyclopedia of Bioethics,* ed. Warren T. Reich (New York: Free Press, 1878); and Martin Pernick, "A Calculus of Suffering: Pain, Anesthesia and Utilitarian Professionalism in 19th-Century American Medicine," (Ph.D. diss., Columbia University, 1978), 1–17.

3. See Pernick, "A Calculus," 112–71.

4. Megali Larson, *The Rise of Professionalism* (Berkeley: University of California Press, 1977), 133.

5. Regina Morantz-Sanchez, "Making Women Modern: Middle Class Women and Health Reform in the 19th-Century America," *Journal of Social History* 10 (Summer 1977): 500.

6. Phrase first used by Daniel Scott Smith in "Family Limitation, Sexual Control and Domestic Feminism in Victorian America" in M. Hartman and L. Banner, eds., *Class Consciousness Raised; New Perspectives on the History of Women* (New York: Harper & Row, 1974). See also Kathryn Kish Sklar, *Catherine Beecher,* (New Haven, CT: Yale University Press, 1973), and Nancy Cott, *The Bonds of Womanhood* (New Haven, CT: Yale University Press, 1977) for examples of the argument.

7. Regina Morantz-Sanchez, "The 'Connecting Link': The case for the Woman Doctor in 19th-Century America," in *Sickness and Health in America,* eds. R. Numbers and J. Leavitt, (Madison: University of Wisconsin Press, 1978).

8. "On the Education of Women Physicians" [1860], Elizabeth Blackwell Papers, Box 59, Library of Congress, Washington, D.C.; Ann Preston, *Valedictory Address* (Philadelphia, 1858), 9; Elizabeth Blackwell, *Medicine as a Profession for Women* (New York: 1860), 10–11.

9. Harriot Hunt's remarks in *Proceedings of the Women's Rights Convention, October, 1851* (Boston: 1852). Price, "The Necessity for Women Physicians," Medical College of Pennsylvania Archives 1871; Saur, "Physicians and Their Duties," MCP, 1871.

10. See James J. Walsh, "Women in the Medical World," *New York Medical Journal* 96 (1912): 1324–28; Morantz-Sanchez, "Connecting Link," 117.

11. The five "regular" schools were the Woman's Medical College of Pennsylvania (1850 to present); New England Female Medical College (1856–73), which merged with the homeopathic Boston University; Woman's Medical College of Chicago

(1870–1902); Woman's Medical College of Baltimore (1882–1909). See Morantz-Sanchez, "Connecting Link," 117.

12. See Regina Markell Morantz, "Women Physicians, Co-education and the Struggle for Professional Standards in 19th-Century Medical Education" (Paper delivered at Berkshire Conference, Mount Holyoke College, South Hadley, MA, August 1978); Martin Kaufman, "The Admission of Women to 19th-Century Medical Societies," *Bulletin of the History of Medicine* 50 (Summer 1976): 251–59.

13. W. W. Parker, M.D., "Woman's Place in the Christian World: Superior Morally, Inferior Mentally to Man—Not Qualified for Medicine or Law—the Contrariety and Harmony of the Sexes," *Transactions of the Medical Society of the State of Virginia* (1892): 86–107. See also Mary Roth Walsh, *"Doctors Wanted: No Women Need Apply," Sexual Barriers in the Medical Profession, 1835–1975* (New Haven, CT: Yale University Press, 1977); and Gloria Melnick Moldow, "The Gilded Age, Promise and Disillusionment: Women Doctors and the Emergence of the Professional Middle Class, Washington, D.C., 1870–1900" (Ph.D. diss., University of Maryland, 1980).

14. See *Boston Medical and Surgical Journal* 111 (1884): 90; ibid. 40 (1849): 505; ibid. 89 (1873): 23.

15. Edmund Andrews, M.D., "The Surgeon," *Chicago Medical Examiner* 2 (1861): 587–98, quoted in Pernick, "A Calculus," 131; Newspaper clipping, n.d., Chadwick Scrapbook, Countway Library, Boston, Mass., cited in Walsh, *"Doctors Wanted,"* 139. For a good discussion of doctors' fears of feminization, see Pernick, "A Calculus," *passim,* and Walsh, *"Doctors Wanted,"* 135–46.

16. E. H. Clarke, *Sex in Education: A Fair Chance for Girls* (Boston: 1873), 23; also Horatio Storer, "Letter of Resignation," *Boston Medical and Surgical Journal* 75 (1866): 191–92.

17. Clarke, *Sex in Education,* 41.

18. M. Carey Thomas, "Present Tendencies in Women's College and University Education," *Educational Review* 25 (1908): 68.

19 Mary Putnam Jacobi, *The Question of Rest for Women during Menstruation* (New York: 1877); Emily F. Pope, M.D., and Emma Call, M.D., *The Practice of Medicine by Women in the United States* (Boston: 1881), 7.

20. See, for example, Elizabeth C. Underhill, M.D., "The Effect of College Life on the Health of Women Students," *Woman's Medical Journal* 22 (February 1912): 31–33; Mary E. B. Ritter, M.D., "Health of University Girls," *California State Medical Journal* 1 (1902–3): Clelia Mosher, M.D., "Some of the Causal Factors in the Increased Height of College Women," *Journal of the American Medical Association* 81 (August 1923): 535–38; Elizabeth R. Thelburg, "College Education a Factor in the Physical Life of Women," *Transactions of the Alumnae Association of the Woman's Medical College of Pennsylvania* (1899): 73–87. See also Virginia Drachman, "Women Doctors and the Women's Medical Movement: Feminism and Medicine, 1850–1895," (Ph.D. diss., State University of New York at Buffalo, 1976) for a somewhat different perspective.

21. M. Carey Thomas, *The Opening of the Johns Hopkins Medical School to Women,* pamphlet reprinted from *The Century Magazine* (February 1891), Sophia Smith College Collection, Northampton, MA, box labeled "Physicians U.S."; Mary Putnam Jacobi, "Social Aspects of the Readmission of Women into the Medical Profession," *Papers and Letters Presented at the First Woman's Congress of the Association for the Advancement of Woman* (New York: 1874), 174.

22. See, for example, Josephine Baker's comments about Emily Blackwell and other women faculty at the New York Infirmary in her Fighting for Life (New York: Macmillan, 1959), 34–44; and Emily Dunning Barringer's remarks in her *Bowery*

to Bellevue (New York: W. W. Norton, 1950), 60–61, and Jacobi, "Social Aspects," 80–81. See also the correspondence between Elizabeth Blackwell and Eliza Mosher in Mosher Papers, Michigan Historical Collections, University of Michigan, Ann Arbor, MI.

23. For a thoughtful discussion of feminist thought on the subject of marriage, see William Leach, *True Love and Perfect Union: The Feminist Reform of Sex and Society* (New York: Basic Books, 1980), 38–132.

24. Georgiana Glenn, "Are Women as Capable of Becoming Physicians as Men," *The Clinic* 9 (1875): 243–45; Jacobi, "Inaugural Address Delivered at the Women's Medical College of the New York Infirmary," 1880, *Chicago Medical Journal & Examiner* 42 (1881): 580.

25. Eliza Mosher to sister, April 17, 1887, Mosher Papers, Michigan Historical Collections. Frances A. Rutherford, M.D., "The New Force in Medicine and Surgery," *Proceedings of the Michigan State Medical Society* (1893), 4.

26. See Annie S. Daniel, "A Cautious Experiment," *Woman's Medical Journal* 47 (July 1940): 201; Elizabeth Blackwell, *Pioneer Work in Opening the Medical Profession to Women* (New York: 1895), 227; "Pioneer Medical Women of Cleveland," *Journal of American Medical Women's Association* 6 (May 1951): 186–89; Edna H. Nelson, *The Women and Children's Hospital,* pamphlet reprinted from *Hospital Council Bulletin* 10 (January 1941), Radcliffe Women's Archives, Radcliffe College, Cambridge, MA, hereinafter cited as RWA. Lillian Welsh, *Reminiscences of Thirty Years in Baltimore* (Baltimore: Norman, Remington, 1925), 48–61, for a description of the medical social work carried out by the women physicians at the Evening Dispensary for Working Women. On the New England Hospital for Women and Children, see Regina Markell Morantz and Sue Zschoche, "Professionalism, Feminism, and Gender Roles: A Comparative Study of Nineteenth-Century Medical Therapeutics," *Journal of American History* 67 (December 1980): 568–88.

27. Garrigue to Blackwell, December 21, 1899, Blackwell Manuscripts, RWA; Jacobi, "Woman in Medicine," in *Woman's Work in America,* ed. Annie Nathan Meyer (New York: 1891), 171.

Will There Be a Monument?

Six Pioneer Women Doctors Tell Their Own Stories

RUTH J. ABRAM

THE only medical degree Harriot Hunt (1805–75) possessed was an honorary one from the Woman's Medical College of Pennsylvania. Yet because she was the first woman to apply to Harvard Medical School and because she devoted her life from the earliest days of her medical practice in 1835 to her death in 1875 to the cause of women in medicine, she has earned the title of "mother of the American woman physician." The story of woman's entry into the medical profession, therefore, begins with her.

The first of two daughters born to shipbuilder Joab Hunt and Kezia Wentworth Hunt, Harriot was educated in her native Boston at progressive private schools for girls. Shortly before her father's death in 1827, she opened such a school herself. The grieving family was soon further burdened when Harriot's sister, Sarah, fell ill with what is now thought to have been a tubercular ailment. Desperate after three years of ineffective treatments by regular physicians, the Hunts turned to the British "naturalist" physicians Dr. and Mrs. Mott, under whose ministrations the patient gradually recovered. In 1833, impressed by her sister's recovery Harriot joined Sarah in an apprenticeship with the Motts. With their mother's encouragment, the sisters built up a successful practice, mostly among women and children. Their emphasis on self-knowledge and self-help aroused the ire in some of their male colleagues, as Harriot Hunt remembered:

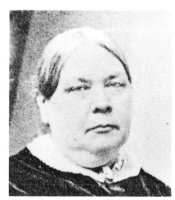

Dr. Harriot K. Hunt, 1805–1875 (c. 1870). The Schlesinger Library, Radcliffe College.

71

1831	1832	1833	1837
Chloroform discovered by Dr. Samuel Guthrie	Cholera epidemic kills 6,000 in New Orleans Boston Lying-In Hospital established	American Anti-Slavery Society founded Davenport invents electric motor	Mount Holyoke Female Seminary founded First antislavery Convention of American Women takes place Electric Telegraph invented

Whenever I had aroused a family to thought on these matters [of self-knowledge], I heard that the attending physician, with few exceptions had said something to this effect—"It is not fitting for women to know about themselves; it makes them nervous!" . . . [One] lady patient [responded,] "Are they not nervous enough through ignorance?"[1]

After her sister's marriage in 1840, Harriot Hunt maintained the practice alone, continuing her advocacy of self-help. In 1843 she brought the principles of her practice—exercise, rest, diet, and hygiene—to wider audiences by organizing the Ladies' Physiological Society, which held regular discussions on health and hygiene.

In 1832, a year before Harriot Hunt began to study medicine, the family of Samuel and Hannah Lane Blackwell arrived in New York from England. Among the eight children and seven adults that formed the family party was eleven-year-old Elizabeth Blackwell (1821–1910). Her father, an active Dissenter, had decided to try his prospects in America after his sugar refinery was destroyed by fire. The ocean voyage did nothing to dampen the family's reform spirits, for soon after their arrival they threw themselves into the abolition movement. Samuel Blackwell's opposition to slavery led him to experiment with beet-sugar refinement to avoid using slave-picked cane. Left in dire economic straits after their father's death in 1838, the older children worked to support and educate the younger ones. At seventeen, Elizabeth organized a private school with her mother and elder sisters; later she taught in Kentucky.

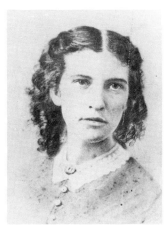

Elizabeth Blackwell as a young girl (c. 1842). ASCWM, MCP.

In 1845, feeling "the want of a more engrossing pursuit," twenty-four-year-old Elizabeth paid a visit to a dying friend. This act of mercy changed the course of Blackwell's life. Fifty years later she remembered it vividly:

My friend died of a painful disease, the delicate nature of which made the methods of treatment a constant suffering to her. She once said to me: ". . . If I could have been treated by a lady doctor, my worst sufferings would have been spared me."

. . . I resolutely tried for weeks to put the idea suggested by my friend away; but it constantly recurred to me.

. . . the idea of winning a doctor's degree gradually assumed the aspect of a great moral struggle, and the moral fight possessed immense attraction for me.[2]

With money saved from her teaching salary, Blackwell began applying to medical schools in Boston, New York, and Philadelphia, all the while ap-

1839	1841	1842	1844
C. W. Pennock invents flexible-tube stethoscope, Philadelphia **Baltimore College of Dental Surgery founded, first in world**	First wagon train to California First university degrees granted to women in U.S.	Dorothea Dix demands humane, specialized care for insane Dr. Crawford Long of Georgia makes first use of ether as general anaesthetic	Dr. Horace Wells demonstrates "laughing gas" (nitrous oxide) American Psychiatric Association founded

pealing to friends for support. Her diary recorded their disappointing responses:

> May 27, 1847—Called on Dr. Jackson . . . I told him I wanted to study medicine. He began to laugh . . . the professors were all opposed to my entrance.

> June 2, 1847—Felt as gloomy as thunder . . . my kindly Quaker adviser, whose private lectures I attended, said to me: "Elizabeth, it is of no use trying. Thee must go to Paris and don masculine attire to gain the necessary knowledge."[3]

Blackwell was particularly discouraged by the reaction of Harriet Beecher Stowe, author of *Uncle Tom's Cabin*:

> Mrs. Beecher Stowe thought, after conversation with Professor Stowe, that my idea was impractible [*sic*]. . . . She also spoke of the strong prejudice which would exist, which I must either crush or be crushed by. I felt a little disappointed at her judgment.[4]

Still, Blackwell persisted, her goal having now assumed the character of a religious calling: "I *knew* that, however insignificant my individual effort might be, it was in a right direction, and in accordance with the great providential ordering of our race's progress."[5]

In October 1847, after months of rejections, Elizabeth Blackwell was accepted by the Geneva Medical College in upstate New York. "With an immense sigh of relief and aspiration of profound gratitude to Providence," Blackwell "instantly accepted the invitation and prepared for the journey."[6]

But her admission had been an accident. Confident that the student body would reject Blackwell's application, the faculty had placed the matter before the young men for a vote. Assuming the request was a joke, the students voted unanimous approval. Two weeks later, Blackwell commenced her studies at Geneva with sober determination.

News of Blackwell's admission to Geneva Medical College spread widely. In Boston, it served to inspire forty-two-year-old Harriot Hunt, now with twelve years of practice behind her, to write a letter of application to Dean Oliver Wendell Holmes of Harvard Medical School. Her application was summarily dismissed as "inexpedient." Not satisfied with this reason, Hunt reapplied on November 12, 1850, closing her letter, "Shall mind, or sex, be

In whatever situation of life a woman is placed from her cradle to her grave, a spirit of obedience and submission, pliability of temper, and humility of mind are required of her.
—A lady, author of *The Young Lady's Book*

The differences between the sexes does not imply inferiority, for it is part of the order of Nature established by Him.
—Mrs. Lydia Sigourney

WILL THERE BE A MONUMENT?

73

1846	1847	1848	1848
Smithsonian Institution founded Sewing machine patented by Elias Howe First demonstration of sulfuric ether, Massachusetts General Hospital	Astronomer Maria Mitchell discovers new comet New York Academy of Medicine founded American Medical Association founded	California Gold Rush begins First woman's rights conference, Seneca Falls, New York First appendectomy performed by Dr. Hancock	Dr. Samuel Gregory founds New England Female Medical College, Boston

recognized in admission to medical lectures?"[7] A month later she received permission to purchase lecture tickets, but was reminded not to assume that this meant she might eventually claim a Harvard degree. In early 1851, however, even this grudging concession was withdrawn, when Harvard's senior class presented the medical faculty with a six-point protest, including the following resolution:

Woman has a head almost too small for intellect but just big enough for love.
— Dr. Charles Meigs

We should give to man cheerfully the curative department and woman the preventive.
— Dr. Harriot Hunt

Resolved, That no woman of true delicacy would be willing in the presence of men to listen to the discussion of the subjects that necessarily come under the consideration of the student of medicine.

Resolved, That we object to having the company of any female forced upon us, who is disposed to unsex herself, and to sacrifice her modesty, by appearing with men in the medical lecture room.

Resolved, That we are not opposed to allowing woman her rights, but do protest against her appearing in places where her presence is calculated to destroy our respect for the modesty and delicacy of her sex.[8]

Faced with this strong opposition, Harvard's trustees passed a resolution specifically prohibiting the admission of women, a policy in force until 1946.

Meanwhile, at Geneva Medical College, Elizabeth Blackwell successfully protested her exclusion from classroom demonstrations, swallowed her embarassment over the examination of female patients in the private rooms of her professors, and withstood the jeers of townspeople. Diary entries during

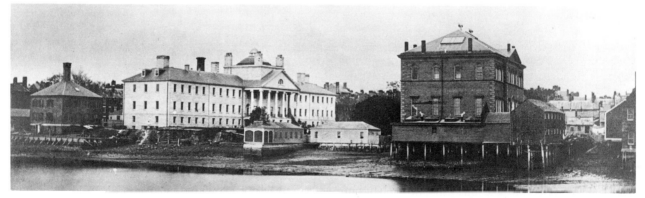

Harvard Medical School (1853). Countway Library of Medicine, Boston.

1850	1851	1852	1853
First National Woman's Rights Convention, Worcester, Massachusetts University of Michigan Medical School founded	*New York Times* first published Maine and Illinois adopt prohibition Harriet Tubman begins slave rescue campaign	*Uncle Tom's Cabin*, by Harriet Beecher Stowe, published American Pharmaceutical Association founded	Hypodermic needle first used for injections

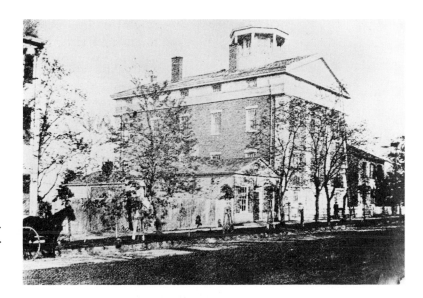

Geneva Medical College (c. 1848).
Courtesy Geneva Historical Society.

this period suggest some of the personal strain of Blackwell's public stead-fastness:

> December 4, 1847—Doctor Webster sent for me to examine a case of a poor woman at his rooms. 'Twas a horrible exposure indecent for any poor woman to be subject to such a torture; she seemed to feel it, poor and ignorant as she was. I felt more than ever the necessity of my mission. But I went home out of spirits, I hardly know why. I felt alone. I must work by myself all life long.[9]

In the summer of 1848, between sessions at Geneva, Blackwell secured practical training at Blockley Almshouse in Philadelphia. Blackwell remembered the experience bitterly:

> The young resident physicians, unlike their chief, were not friendly. When I walked into the wards they walked out. They ceased to write the diagnosis and treatment of patients on the card at the head of each bed, which had hitherto been the custom, thus throwing me entirely on my own resources for clinical study.[10]

Graduating at the top of her class in 1849, Dr. Elizabeth Blackwell, the first American woman to obtain a medical degree, sailed to Europe for two

[We] look to [women] to elevate the profession.
—Dr. Joseph Longshore

WILL THERE BE A MONUMENT?

1854	1855	1855	1857
Republican party formed	Woman's Hospital founded in New York City by Dr. J. Marion Sims Binaural stethoscope invented by Dr. George P. Camman Florence Nightingale	introduces hygienic standards into military hospitals during Crimean War Jews' Hospital founded in New York City Louisiana establishes first state board of health	Louis Pasteur proves that fermentation is caused by living organisms Dred Scott decision

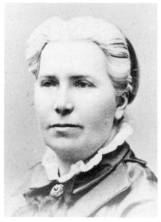

Photograph of Dr. Emily Blackwell. New York Infirmary/Beekman Downtown Hospital.

years of advanced study. There she developed important friendships with supporters of the newly established European women's movement. She returned to New York in 1851 with a renewed commitment, which would be sorely tested during the difficult early years of her practice. She might have drawn some comfort, however, from the knowledge that she would soon have a companion in her pioneering endeavors. In 1848, her sister Emily Blackwell (1826–1910) had enrolled as a private student with John Davis, a demonstrator in anatomy at the Medical College of Cincinnati. Sisterly affection caused Elizabeth to warn her younger sister of the consequences of her choice, saying, "A blank wall of social and professional antagonism faces the woman physician that forms a situation of painful loneliness, leaving her without support, respect or professional counsel."[11] Fortunately for the cause of women in medicine, Emily persisted.

The fourth Blackwell daughter and five years Elizabeth's junior, Emily was eleven years old when her father died. Her early interest in the classics served her well during postgraduate medical training in Europe. Like Elizabeth, Emily saved money for her medical education from her teaching salary, and

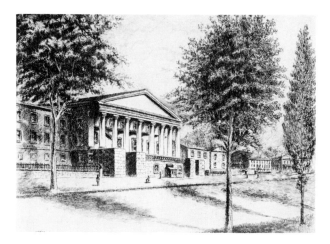

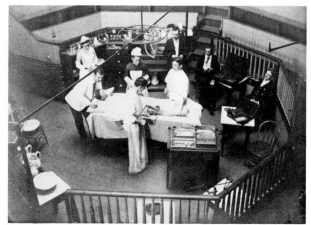

Left: *Painting of exterior of Philadelphia Hospital, Blockley Almshouse, nineteenth century.* Library of the College of Physicians of Philadelphia. Right: *Surgical clinic, Philadelphia Blockley Almshouse.* Library of the College of Physicians of Philadelphia.

1859	1860	1861	1862
Charles Darwin's *Origin of the Species* published Chicago Medical College founded	Bellevue Hospital Medical College founded Dr. Abraham Jacobi founds first children's clinic in U.S. at the New York Medical College	Outbreak of Civil War U.S. Sanitary Commission established Dorothea Dix appointed superintendent of nurses for the Union Army	Emancipation Proclamation frees slaves in rebelling territories Confederacy gives women official nurses status

like Elizabeth, she was willing to struggle to make a place for herself in the decidedly inhospitable medical educational system. Emily Blackwell was rejected by eleven medical schools.

In 1852, Rush Medical College in Chicago broke the pernicious pattern and accepted Emily as a student. Her studies there ended after her first year, however, when the college bowed to pressure from the state medical society and rescinded her admission. Emily spent the summer in New York, gaining practical experience at her sister's side among the poor immigrant women and children who formed the bulk of Elizabeth's practice. In the fall, Emily traveled to Western Reserve Medical College in Cleveland, where she completed her last year of course work. After her March 1854 graduation with honors, Emily left for the continent for two years of additional training. In Edinburgh, London, Paris, Berlin, and Dresden, she observed patient care at hospitals and clinics, experience she would draw upon when she returned to New York to assist her still-struggling sister. Soon, however, the Blackwells would be able to look to trained women physicians outside of the family for support and advice.

Thirty-three-year-old Ann Preston (1813–72) began to read under the Quaker physician Dr. Nathaniel Moseley in 1847, the year Elizabeth Blackwell entered Geneva Medical College. She wished to prepare herself to lecture before ladies' groups on health and hygiene, subjects Preston might have developed an interest in during a childhood darkened by the deaths of two sisters and the invalidism of her mother.

The second of nine children born to Quaker minister Amos Preston and Margaret Smith Preston, Ann was educated in Quaker schools until her mother's illness required her to take over the care of the household. Encouraged by her progressive family, she participated in the abolition and temperance movements and was an early supporter of women's rights.

Upon completing her two-year apprenticeship with Dr. Moseley, Preston determined to acquire a medical degree. She applied to four local medical colleges, but was rejected by all of them.

In Philadelphia, home to a large Quaker community with enlightened views about women's rights, more than one physician had accepted a female student. Frustrated at their inability to secure places for their students in regular medical schools, a group of these doctors decided to found a medical school expressly for women. Dr. Joseph Longshore, whose niece Hannah was also studying medicine privately, took the lead in obtaining a charter. Businessman

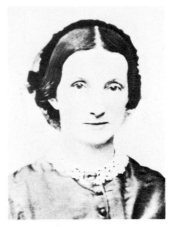

Dr. Ann Preston, 1813–1872 (c. 1850). ASCWM, MCP.

WILL THERE BE A
MONUMENT?

77

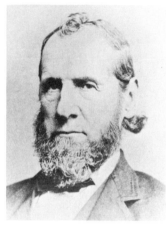

Dr. Joseph Longshore, 1809–1879, one of the founders of the Woman's Medical College of Pennsylvania. ASCWM, MCP.

William Mullen paid the rent on rooms in a house on Arch Street, which became the college's first home.

On October 12, 1850, vowing to provide a medical education "inferior to none," the founders opened the doors of the Woman's Medical College of Pennsylvania, the first regular medical college for women in the world with a student body of forty (Ann Preston among them) and a faculty of six.

On December 30, 1851, the friends and families of Ann Preston and seven other graduates gathered at Philadelphia's Musical Fund Hall. As fifty policemen stood guard against a threatened disruption by male medical students, Dr. Longshore used the occasion of his commencement address to issue a challenge:

We have all been engaged in a new, but momentous enterprize. We have met alike the frowns and prejudices of the community, and labored hand in hand to sustain our institutions against powerful opposing influences. . . .

. . . [The] community will expect as *much,* nay, *more* of you, than of your

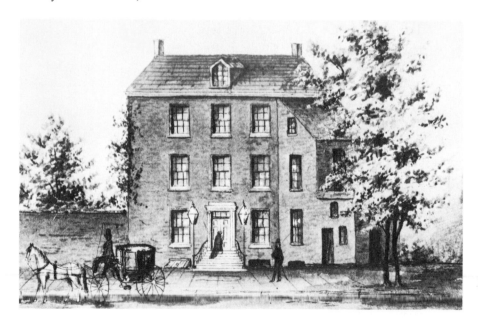

Left: *The Woman's Medical College of Pennsylvania, original location, Arch Street, Philadelphia (c. 1850).* ASCWM, MCP.

Opposite: *First president and faculty, Woman's Medical College of Pennsylvania (c., 1850).* ASCWM, MCP.

1865	1866	1867	1868
Dr. Joseph Lister disinfects wounds with carbolic acid and otherwise initiates antiseptic surgery	Metropolitan Health Board established, New York City	Bellevue Hospital founds "out patient" department	Fourteenth Amendment grants blacks citizenship New England Suffrage Association formed Presbyterian Hospital founded in New York City

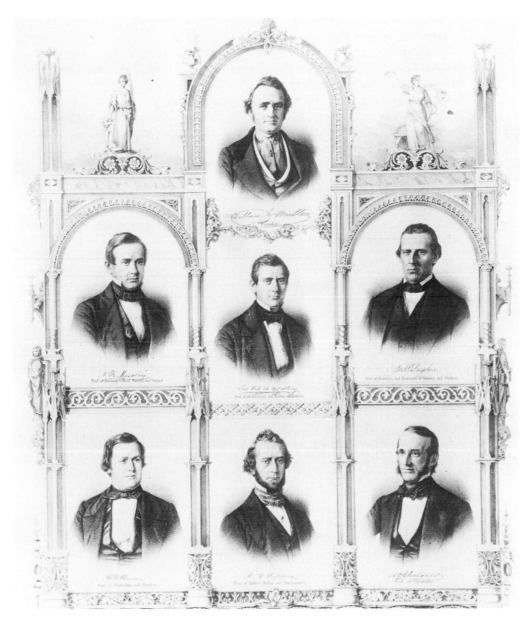

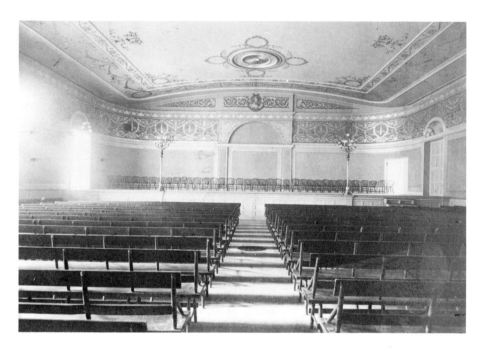

Interior of Music Fund Hall, Philadelphia, where the first commencement exercises of the Woman's Medical College of Pennsylvania took place. ASCWM, MCP.

professional brethren. And the question now to be settled to put the opposers of female medical education forever at rest, is, whether woman can here sustain herself or not. . . . Are you prepared to make the effort? . . . [Your friends] are all, all looking to you and to your future conduct and success with feelings of most intense interest.

. . . Do not, because you are *women* regard yourselves as inferior. . . .[12]

All professions need the two formative forces of nature— the positive and negative, the masculine and feminine . . .
—Dr. Mark Kerr

Dr. Harriot Hunt in Boston and doctors Emily and Elizabeth Blackwell in New York had provided important role models. Now, with the establishment of a medical college for women, American women had their first certain opportunity to obtain regular medical school training. If the movement was to succeed, a supportive network had to be developed. Ann Preston took the first step. In the winter of 1851, Preston journeyed to New York to visit Elizabeth Blackwell. Returned from Europe, Blackwell was in despair over her inability to attract patients. Looking back on that bleak period, Blackwell wrote:

SEND US A LADY PHYSICIAN

80

1872	1873	1873	1874
American Public Health Association founded Morrill Wyman offers first description of hay fever, Cambridge, Massachusetts	U.S. receives 459,803 immigrants Great Depression Woman's Christian Temperance Union founded First national conference of women ministers	Bellevue Hospital founds nursing school	A. T. Still founds osteopathy in Kansas Billroth discovers streptococci and staphylococci University of Pennsylvania establishes a university hospital

> I took good rooms in University Place, but patients came very slowly to consult me. I had no medical companionship, the profession stood aloof, and society was distrustful of the innovation . . . and my pecuniary position was a source of constant anxiety. . . .
>
> . . . Ill-natured gossip as well as insolent letters came to me.[13]

In an 1853 letter to her sister, Blackwell confided, "It *is* hard, with no support but a high purpose, to live against every species of social opposition. . . . I *should* like a little fun now and then. Life is altogether too sober."[14]

Elizabeth Blackwell would remember Ann Preston's inspiring visit for the rest of her life.

> On a wild snowy winter morning, a delicate, refined Quaker lady, called at my consultation room, to tell me about the movement she was engaged in, for the establishment of a thoroughly organized Medical College for Women in Philadelphia—it was Miss Ann Preston. . . . The courage and hope of that fragile lady, who came to me out of the wild snow storm, was an omen of success. I felt sure that she would succeed.[15]

After graduation, Ann Preston commenced her series of lectures on physiology and the laws of life and health for ladies. As she explained in an 1853 letter to a friend, she was encouraged by her reception: "My success has been encouraging. I find generous men and noble women ready to assist and encourage me . . . all recognizing that female physicians are a want of the age. . . . There is a 'good time' coming. . . ."[16]

The following year, Ann Preston was appointed professor of physiology and hygiene at the Woman's Medical College of Pennsylvania. That same year the college awarded Harriot Hunt an honorary degree, and Elizabeth Blackwell opened the New York Dispensary for Poor Women and Children in a single room in an immigrant neighborhood near Tompkins Square.

Blackwell explained the purposes and policies of the dispensary in its first annual report:

> The design of this institution is to give poor women an opportunity of consulting physicians of their own sex.
>
> . . . The dispensary has been regularly opened through the year, on Monday, Wednesday, and Friday afternoons, at 3 o'clock. Over 200 poor women have received medical aid.

To enlighten [women], to teach them the duty they owe to themselves to their families, to posterity . . . is your particular province.
—Dr. Ellwood Harvey

There is room and need [in the medical profession] for both male and female. The character of the profession will be exalted by a blending of masculine and feminine virtues. —Dr. Edwin Fussell

WILL THERE BE A MONUMENT?

81

1875	1875	1876	1878
Civil Rights Act guarantees blacks rights London Medical School for Women founded Dr. S. Weir Mitchell introduces "Rest Cure" Lydia Pinkham produces "Vegetable Compound, a	positive cure for all . . . complaints"	The great Centennial Exposition, Philadelphia Alexander Graham Bell patents the telephone	Robert Koch develops technique for staining and identifying bacteria Thomas Edison invents incandescent bulb Dr. Marion J. Sims performs first gall bladder operation

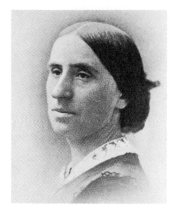

Dr. Marie Zakrzewska, 1829– 1902 (c. 1860). Sophia Smith Collection, Smith College.

With all patients, the necessity of cleanliness, ventilation, and judicious diet have been strongly urged . . . the best methods of seeking employment have been pointed out, suitable charities occasionally recommended, and pecuniary aid sometimes rendered. . . .

It is the hope of the founders of this charity to make it eventually a hospital for women and a school for the education of nurses.[17]

Together with other supporters, Elizabeth Blackwell in New York and Ann Preston in Pennsylvania would pave the way for generations of women in the medical profession. In far away Germany, a circular distributed by the Woman's Medical College of Pennsylvania attracted another to their band. Her name was Marie Zakrzewska (Zak-shek-ska), chief midwife and professor of midwives at Berlin's Charité Hospital.

Born in Berlin, Marie Elizabeth Zakrzewska (1829–1902) was the eldest of five daughters of Martin Ludwig Zakrzewska and Frederika C. W. Urban. Her father was a Prussian army pensioner who had been dismissed from active service for his liberal views. Her mother, a practicing midwife, introduced Marie to the profession. After two years as a private student of Dr. Joseph Schmidt of the School for Midwives at Charité Hospital, Zakrzewska enrolled in the school, graduating in 1851. In 1852, with the backing of her mentor, she was appointed chief midwife and professor at the hospital's School for Midwives. With Dr. Schmidt's death a few hours after her appointment, Zakrzewska lost her main ally. Faced with growing opposition from jealous colleagues at the hospital, she resigned from her post and departed for America in hopes that a country in which a woman's medical college thrived would be a good place to realize her dream of founding her own hospital.

Arriving in New York in 1853 with her younger sister, speaking only German, Zakrzewska sought support from her family's former physician, Dr. Reisig. His patronizing response was Zakrzewska's first indication that the climate for women doctors in America was not what she had hoped: "[Dr. Reisig] informed me that female physicians were of the lowest rank. [But] he said that . . . if I were willing to serve as a nurse . . . he was just then in need of a good one."[18]

Instead, Zak (as Zakrzewska came to be known in America) supported herself and her younger sister by establishing a knitting enterprise. Entries in her journal concerning the women's medical movement suggest the depth of her determination. The most important entry was dated May 15, 1854:

SEND US A LADY PHYSICIAN

On the same morning, I saw Dr. Elizabeth Blackwell—and from this call of the 15th of May, 1854, I date my new life in America. . . .

I cannot comprehend how Dr. Blackwell could ever have taken so deep an interest in me. . . . Yet she did. . . .

She told me of her plan of founding a hospital—the long-cherished idea of my life—and said that she had opened a little dispensary of the 1st of May, two weeks before . . . and she invited me to come and assist her.

She insisted that first of all I should learn English, and she offered to give me lessons twice a week and also to make efforts to enable me to enter a college to acquire the title of "M. D." . . .

The cordiality with which she welcomed me as a co-worker, I can never describe or forget. . . . [A]ll the days of disappointment were instantly forgotten.[19]

If woman's exertions and charities were confined *to [the home and family,] where would be the teachers of the land?* —Dr. Ann Preston

Blackwell was equally stirred, confiding to her diary: "I have at last found a student in whom I can take a great deal of interest. . . . There is true stuff in her, and I shall do my best to bring it out. She must obtain a medical degree. . . ."[20]

In the fall of 1854, Blackwell arranged for Zak's entry into Western Reserve Medical College, from which Emily Blackwell had recently graduated. She also arranged for a scholarship and temporary housing at the home of Cleveland suffragist Caroline Severance, through whom Zak soon met Harriot Hunt.

In spite of this support, Zak's experience in medical school was difficult. She was spurned by the guests at her boarding house and discouraged by some openly hostile professors. A students' petition against the admission of female students succeeded in barring further female admissions for the next twenty-five years.

Through all this Zak managed to stay her course, mastering English and winning the support of the progressive dean of the college. Shortly before the end of her first term, however, she received a devastating blow in the form of a letter from her father in Germany:

Talk about medicine being the appropriate sphere of man and his alone? With tenfold more plausibility and reason might we say, it is the appropriate sphere of woman, and hers alone. —Sarah Hale

My father denounced my leaving my sisters, my despising the sphere of women, and my entering upon a field which so entirely belonged to men; . . . After reading this letter . . . I retired to my room almost in despair.

. . . I resolved to follow my father's advice and give up man's sphere, and offer myself as one of the missionaries to the [Cherokee] Indians.[21]

WILL THERE BE A
MONUMENT?

83

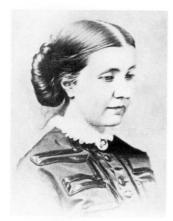

Dr. Lucy E. Sewall, 1837–1890 (c. 1862). Sophia Smith Collection, Smith College.

None need tell [woman] . . . that the work is unsuited to your womanly nature. The contradiction comes not only from your observation of society, but from the deeps of your own souls.

—Dr. Ann Preston

SEND US A LADY PHYSICIAN

84

Friends in Cleveland reminded the distraught student of her special obligation to Elizabeth Blackwell, and a stern letter from that lady persuaded Zak to deny her father and continue her studies. Visits that summer with Blackwell in New York and Hunt in Boston bolstered her flagging spirits, and in March of 1856, Zak proudly received her medical degree, the commencement exhortation to "go out and do honor" to her profession ringing in her ears.

So it was that in the spring of 1856, Elizabeth Blackwell was joined by two women colleagues—Dr. Emily Blackwell, newly returned from Europe, and Dr. Marie Zakrzewska.

Zak's first order of business in New York was to locate and rent a suitable office. Years later Zak recalled how difficult this was:

I investigated everywhere . . . signs announced "Parlor to let for a physician."
. . . But as soon as it was learned that it was a woman physician who desired the office, I was denied. . . .
. . . The name of "Madame Restelle" [*sic*] was on everyone's tongue as typifying the "female physician." She was then the leading abortionist. . . .[22]

Finally, Zak accepted Elizabeth Blackwell's offer to live at her home, now bursting with three generations of the famous Blackwell reformers.[23]

In spite of a decided shortage of patients, the three doctors, Emily and Elizabeth Blackwell and Zak, began to work in earnest toward the realization of their common dream: to found a hospital run by women expressly for women.

The indefatigable Zak took on the job of fundraising in Boston. There she stopped at the home of Lucy Sewall, who, long after she had completed medical school and taken her place in the leadership of the women's medical movement, admitted to Zak her initial doubts. While Zak waited in the downstairs parlor on that day, Sewall did some detective work upstairs. Zak recounted the story with forgiving humor: "[She] examined my cloak, bonnet, and gloves in order to find out whether they were neat and respectable, she feeling a great uncertainty as to whether a regularly graduated and practicing woman physician could attend the minor details of proper habiliment."[24]

Back in New York, the Blackwell sisters encountered a much stronger variety of social opposition in their attempts to win supporters and otherwise make arrangements for the opening of the hospital. Warnings that "no one would let a house for the purpose, that female doctors would be looked upon

1889	1889	1890	1892
Jane Addams and Ellen Starr open Hull House Second great flu epidemic Von Mehring and Minkowski prove that the pancreas secretes insulin, preventing	diabetes Sterile surgical gloves introduced Mayo Clinic opens in Rochester, Minnesota	Daughters of the American Revolution founded U.S. Public Health Service begins inspection of immigrants Global influenza epidemics	People's Party (Populists) founded Ida Wells-Barnett begins antilynching campaign Iron and Steel workers strike First automatic telephone switchboard introduced

with so much suspicion that the police would interfere; that if deaths occurred their death certificates would not be recognized"[25] failed to dissuade them. Ultimately, Zak's fundraising skills; the moral support of numerous men and women in Philadelphia, Boston, and New York; and the determination of the Blackwell sisters won the day: on May 1, 1857, the New York Infirmary for Women and Children opened its doors. Just as the opening of the Woman's Medical College of Pennsylvania had guaranteed women the opportunity to receive a medical education, the opening of the New York Infirmary—the first hospital ever run entirely by women—guaranteed women the opportunity to gain the practical experience so necessary for complete training.

The Reverend Henry Ward Beecher, Quaker Dr. William Elder, and the Reverend Dr. Tyng spoke at the opening ceremonies, the patrons having rejected Zak's suggestion that Elizabeth Blackwell address the crowd, fearing Blackwell would speak "like a Woman's Rights woman."[26]

The infirmary opened at 64 Bleeker Street with Dr. Zakrzewska as resident physician and Dr. Emily Blackwell in charge of the surgical practice. Zak recalled the physical facilities clearly:

> The front entrance hall was comfortably arranged with settees for the patients to wait their turn. Donations from several wholesale druggists were received, and second-hand furniture suitable for our purposes was cheaply acquired. . . .
>
> The second floor was arranged for two wards, each containing six beds; while the third floor was made into a maternity department, the little hall serving as a sitting room for the physicians. Open coal grate fires provided the only heat throughout the house.
>
> The fourth, or attic, floor contained four rooms. . . . The two large rooms served as sleeping rooms, one for the four students and the other for three servants. One of the small rooms served a similar purpose for the resident physician and one student, while the other was the much needed store and trunk room.[27]

Patient demand for services ran high, but so did criticism and fear. Elizabeth Blackwell remembered how important the support of certain prominent male physicians was in withstanding this prejudice:

> Through a cloud of discouragement and distrust the little medical institution steadily worked its way. . . . The practice of the infirmary, both medical and surgical, was conducted entirely by women; but a board of consulting physicians, men of high standing in the profession, gave it the sanction of their names. Dr. Valentine Mott, Dr. John Watson, Drs. Willard Parker, R. S. Kissam, Isaac E.

The intuitions, observations, sympathies and knowledge of educated and true women must enlarge the common possessions of the professions . . . —Dr. Ann Preston

[Woman] must correct the silly sentimentality which the world has manifested for her sex. She must spurn the spurious gallantry with which she is treated and insist on a standard of treatment . . . in consonance with an advanced civilization. —Dr. Mark Kerr

WILL THERE BE A MONUMENT?

85

1892	1893	1893	1893
Sir William Osler publishes *Principles and Practice of Medicine* George M. Sternberg publishes *A Manual of Bacteriology*	Karl Benz and Henry Ford build their first cars Congress of Jewish women organized (National Congress of Jewish Women) Johns Hopkins Medical	School opens First American chair in pharmacology created at Johns Hopkins Theobold Smith proves disease can be transmitted by insects Lillian Wald founds	Henry Street Settlement Visiting Nurse Service

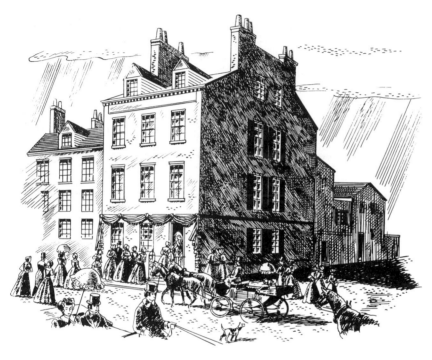

Artist's rendering of activity outside the original site of the New York Infirmary, Bleecker Street (1857). New York Infirmary/Beekman Downtown Hospital.

Taylor, and George P. Camman were the earliest medical friends of the infirmary.[28]

[Women] will be so clothed with the attributes of refined womanhood, [they] will dignify the profession.
—Dr. Mary J. Scarlett

SEND US A LADY PHYSICIAN

In the infirmary's first year relatives of a woman who died in childbirth surrounded the hospital. Zak remembered their threatening mood: "An immense crowd collected, filling the block between us and Broadway, hooting and yelling and trying to push in the doors. . . ."[29] Armed with pickaxes and shovels, they demanded admission, shouting that the female physicians were killing women with cold water.

The neighborhood police, now accustomed to escorting the hardy women physicians through the night to neighborhood sick beds, saved the day. According to Zak, "they commanded silence and ordered the crowd to disperse, telling them that they knew the doctors in that hospital treated the patients in the best possible way, and that no doctor could keep everybody from dying sometime."[30]

1893	1894	1895	1896
Bureau of Immigration founded First polio epidemic in U.S.	Diphtheria treatment developed Wilhelm Roentgen discovers X-rays	Supreme Court approves "separate but equal" doctrine National Association of Colored Women founded Nurses Associated Alumnae formed (American Nurses	Association) X-ray treatment used for first time Antityphoid innoculation introduced

The infirmary's beds were filled again before the month was out and soon the hospital staff—with the doctors Blackwell and Zak attending the dispensary two mornings a week and four students from the Woman's Medical College of Pennsylvania serving as interns, apothecaries, and nurses—was hard put to handle the flow of patients. The daily schedule, as described in Zak's diary, was exhausting:

At 5:30 A.M., I started in an omnibus for the wholesale market, purchasing provisions for the week, and at 8:00, I was back to breakfast. . . .

After breakfast, I made my visit to the patients in the house with two of the students. . . . Then a confinement case arrived and I attended to her. . . . After this, I descended into the kitchen department, as the provisions had arrived, . . . and I settled the diet for all as far as possible.

I then took another omnibus ride to the wholesale druggist, begging and buying needed articles for the dispensary and the hospital, arriving home at 1:00 P.M., for dinner. This consisted every day of a good soup, the soup meat, potatoes, one kind of well-prepared vegetable, with fruit for dessert. . . .

After dinner, I usually went out to see my private patients, because receiving no compensation I depended upon my earnings for personal needs. On this day,

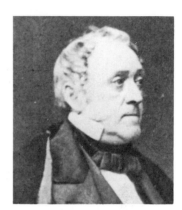

Dr. Valentine Mott, 1785–1865 (c. 1835) NYAM.

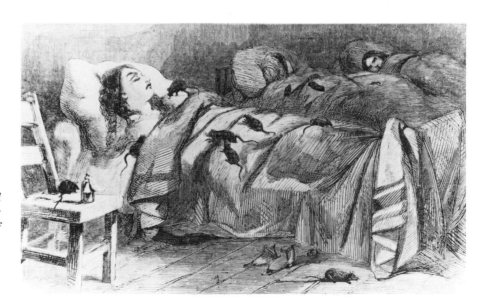

Picture of Bellevue Hospital from Harper's Weekly *(1860). Museum of the city of New York.*

Marie and Pierre Curie discover radium and polonium Epinephrin (adrenalin) isolated by John Jacob Abel of Johns Hopkins	**Carrie Nation begins antisaloon campaign Max Planck formulates quantum theory The American Association of Pathologists and Bacteriologists founded**	**Walter Reed investigates yellow fever in Havana Karl Landsteiner divides blood cells into three groups; makes blood transfusion reliable**

however, I was detained by the confinement case mentioned and could not go out till 5:00 P.M., returning at 7:00 P.M. for tea. This always consisted of bread and butter, tea and sauce or cheese or fresh gingerbread. After making the rounds of the patients in the house, it was 9:00.

Then the students assembled with me. . . . I cutting out towels or pillow cases or other needed articles for the house or the patients, while the students folded or even basted the articles for the sewing machine as they recited their various lessons for the day. After their recital, I gave them verbal instructions in midwifery. We finished the work of the day by 11:30, as I never allowed any one to be out of bed after midnight unless detained by a patient.[31]

The physiological peculiarities of woman . . . cannot fail frequently to interfere with the regular discharge of her duties as physician . . .
—Discussion in Philadelphia County Medical Society

The infirmary expanded rapidly, and soon a larger building was required. In August 1859, Blackwell reported that a "spacious house, 126 Second Avenue, was purchased and adapted to the use of hospital and dispensary, with accommodation for several students. . . . [W]e carried on the rapidly growing work of the infirmary with the aid of intelligent graduates from Philadelphia, who came to us for practical instruction in medicine."[32]

Victorian women physicians took their roles as society's guardians seriously. It is not surprising then that the New York Infirmary was the first hospital to establish a tenement service. And if the choice of America's second black woman physician to head up the service seemed novel to Elizabeth Blackwell, it was not reflected in her matter-of-fact report:

The study of medicine has but strengthened . . . womanly feelings.
—Dr. Emeline H. Cleveland

We established [the post of] sanitary visitor . . . whose special duty it was to give simple, practical instruction to poor mothers on the management of infants and the preservation of the health of their families. An intelligent young coloured physician, Dr. Cole, who was one of our resident assistants, carried on this work with tact and care. Experience of its results serve to show that the establishment of such a department would be a valuable addition to every hospital.[33]

Rebecca Cole (1846–1922) was the first black graduate of the Woman's Medical College of Pennsylvania and the second regularly trained black woman physician in the United States. Dr. Ann Preston had served as her preceptor. After serving at the New York Infirmary, Cole returned to Philadelphia as assistant director of the Women's Directory, a charitable organization that provided free medical and legal services to poor women. In her fifty years of active practice, Dr. Cole also worked in Columbia, South Carolina, and Washington, D.C.

SEND US A LADY PHYSICIAN

88

The establishment of these two important institutions—the Woman's Medical College of Pennsylvania and the New York Infirmary for Women and Children—laid the foundation for a separate women's sphere. Leaders of both these institutions were in frequent contact with one another, as were the students they trained. Even at this early stage, however, the movement leaders pressed toward their ultimate goal—entry into the male medical establishment.

Anxious to broaden the opportunities for practical study open to her students, Ann Preston petitioned the Philadelphia medical schools to allow women to attend their clinical lectures. When she was refused, she chided the recalcitrant administrators, pointing out that the women had asked for access to the clinics only "for the purpose of qualifying themselves to practice, more intelligently, the art of healing."[34] Preston, however, was undaunted by their refusal. She believed these trials would be temporary, explaining to a friend in 1855, "It will not long be thus; our day will come; we will work in faith, and bide our time."[35]

In 1856, Preston's repeated petitions were successful; she and a group of students were allowed to purchase tickets to clinical lectures at Philadelphia Hospital's Blockley Almshouse. But Dr. Hayes Agnew, professor at Jefferson Medical College, fought back. When his display of a nude male patient failed to drive the women away, he successfully appealed to the hospital board to bar women from further attendance.

In 1858, the fledgling movement for women in medicine sustained an even greater blow, when the Board of Censors of the Philadelphia County Medical Society formally ostracized the Woman's Medical College, making impossible the admission of women to public teaching clinics or membership in any medical society, including the American Medical Association:

> The Censors respectfully report that they would recommend the members of the regular profession to withhold from the faculties and graduates of the female medical colleges, all countenance and support, and that they cannot, consistently with sound medical ethics, consult or hold professional medical intercourse with their professors or alumnae.[36]

In vain, the medical societies in Lancaster and Montgomery counties passed dissenting resolutions, calling the Board of Censor's action "not only premature, ill-advised and injudicious, but also [evidence] of reprehensible prejudice and illiberality."[37] The prominent Quaker physician Hiram Corson was at the fore of these and other campaigns against sexism in the profession throughout his lifetime.

Clearly a long and bitter battle would have to be waged in order to gain access to Philadelphia's abundant clinical facilities. Preston soon realized that the Woman's Medical College would have to open up its own clinics in order to provide students with the necessary practical training.

Back in New York, the New York Infirmary was prospering; its financial condition had improved significantly since its shaky opening. Marie Zakrzewska had earned enough money from her private practice to repay her debts. These factors, along with a natural desire to make her own mark, precipitated Zak's decision to leave the infirmary. In June of 1859, she left

Medical literature and medical feeling . . . need the refining and ennobling influences that . . . true woman . . . give [sic]. —Dr. Ann Preston

I can see no good reasons why women should not be regarded as legally . . . members of the medical profession. —Dr. Harding

This war against women is beneath the dignity of a learned society of scientific men. —Dr. James King

WILL THERE BE A MONUMENT?

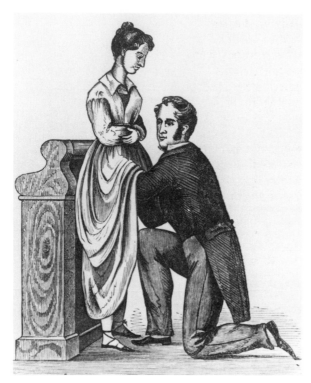

Male midwifery as illustrated in Samuel Gregory's Medical Morals *(c. 1852)* New York Academy of Medicine.

New York to accept the position of professor of obstetrics and diseases of women and to become director of a proposed clinical department at New England Female Hsopital and Medical College in Boston.

Again Zak's memoirs recall her father's angry response to her career advancement:

He now became really distressing to me because his conviction was that whether I succeeded or not I was disgracing the family, and German womanhood in general, by accepting a position which caused my name to come prominently before the public.

I finally felt that I must write a strong and decided letter to him, requesting him either to stop writing to me altogether or else to preserve silence as to his judgment of me and my actions. This letter arrived in Berlin at a time when he was ill . . . and he died a few days later. . . . I never knew whether he read my letter or not.[38]

The New England Female Medical College had been founded in 1848 by the controversial Dr. Samuel Gregory, who for years after graduating from Yale toured the country lecturing on such topics as mesmerism, phrenology, and licentiousness. His reputation was established after his pamphlet "Facts and Important Information for Young Men on the Self-Indulgence of the Sexual Appetite" sold forty-two thousand copies. Believing that male midwives threatened female virtue, Gregory decided to provide female midwives with formal training. A graduate of an "irregular" medical school, Gregory maintained a hostility to the established profession that was repaid in kind.

Zak's pleasure over assuming this position soon gave way to despair, as ignorant trustees and Dr. Gregory blocked her every attempt to improve the school. Her requests for thermometers, microscopes, and test tubes were denied on the grounds that these were "new-fangled European notions."

Zak remembered her frustration when a trustee, threatened by her scientific approach, said, "We need a doctor . . . who knows when a patient has a fever, or what ails her, without a microscope. We need practical persons in our American life."[39]

When her own students resisted Zak's pleas that they obtain practical training, the concerned teacher tried to understand, reminding herself that the "prevailing custom in even the best medical schools [was purely theoretical, and] students were expected to procure their practical training at the hands of their private preceptors . . . training [which was] . . . liable to be a will-o'-the-wisp."[40]

The promiscuous intermingling of the sexes in our schools, I utterly repudiate. I say, let her stay home and put on an apron and attend to her children. —Dr. Henry Gibbons

In 1861, unable to surmount her opposition and unwilling to be a part of an institution that turned out ignorant and ill-prepared graduates, Zak resigned, immediately turning her attention to the founding of the New England Hospital for Women and Children, an institution that *would* meet her high standards for medical care.

Encouraged by highly esteemed male Boston physicians, including doctors S. Cotting, Walter Channing, H. I. Bowditch, Henry E. Clark, and S. Cabot, Zak decided to seek membership in the Massachusetts Medical Society. With earnest expectations Zak prepared for the examinations and applied for permission to take them. Unfortunately, her supporters, though influential in the Society, were unable to outvote her opponents. Her application was dismissed by reason of her sex.

Zak again applied and was rejected in 1864. (It was not until 1884, when she was overy fifty years old and had twenty-six years of practice behind her, that Zak was finally invited to take the Society examinations. She refused the offer as condescending.)

In the midst of these trials and triumphs in Boston, Philadelphia, and New York, the Civil War erupted. Elizabeth Blackwell remembered the strong effect the war's outbreak had on her and the women reformers with whom

It seems to be [men's] ambition to cure disease and very seldom do any of them think it worth their while to teach their patients how to prevent a return of their maladies.
—Dr. Amanda Price

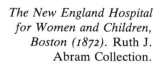

The New England Hospital for Women and Children, Boston (1872). Ruth J. Abram Collection.

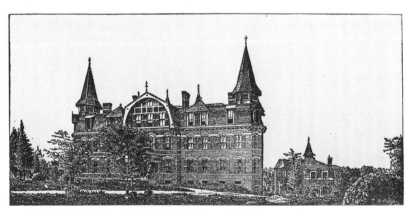

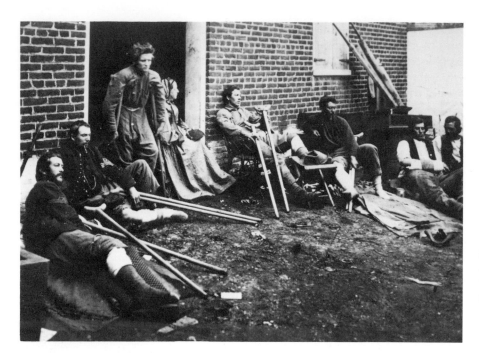

Civil War wounded with Sanitary Commission nurse at Fredricksburg, Virginia Depot where crutches were distributed (1864). Burns Archive.

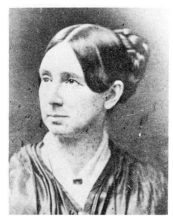

Dorothea Dix, 1802–1887 (c. 1850). The Schlesinger Library, Radcliffe College.

she worked: "In the full tide of our medical activity in New York, . . . the great catastrophe of civil war overwhelmed the country and dominated every other interest." Actively participating in the Ladies' Sanitary Aid Association and the National Sanitary Aid Association, Blackwell and her board of lady managers responded to the desperate cry for help coming from the battlefields by organizing to supply trained nurses to the front lines: "All that could be done in the extreme urgency of the need was to sift out the most promising women . . . put them for a month in training at Bellevue Hospital . . . and send them on for distribution to Miss Dix, who was appointed superintendent of nurses at Washington."[41]

In Boston, Marie Zakrzewska did her part to fill the demand for trained nurses. She and her supporters opened the New England Hospital for Women and Children on July 1, 1862, in the middle of the Civil War. The aims of the institution, Zak explained, were; "1. To provide for women medical aid by competent physicians of their own sex; 2. To assist educated women in the practical study of medicine; 3. To train nurses for the care of the sick."[42] Zak was aided in this endeavor by both Lucy Sewall, who had been among Zak's first students at the New England Female Medical College, and Sewall's father, Samuel Edmund, a distinguished Bostonian.

In Philadelphia, Ann Preston's disappointment over the interruption of classes at the Woman's Medical College of Pennsylvania was tempered by encouraging developments in her goal of building a woman's hospital. She had organized a meeting at the home of the abolitionist and suffrage leader Lucretia Mott, a sister Quaker. Zak, who was a guest speaker at the meeting was struck by Mrs. Mott's reaction to the idea of founding a hospital· "Then thee thinks that a hospital must be connected with the college? . . . We thank thee for thy coming to tell us so, and we promise thee that we shall exert ourselves at once to get a hospital of our own."[43]

Preston lost no time in rallying additional supporters to the cause, approaching, as she explained, "everyone who I thought would give me either money or influence."[44] In September of 1861, the Woman's Hsopital of Philadelphia opened. The hospital's first annual report set forth the institutions' purpose, to provide a retreat where, "without violence to their sensibilities," ladies could receive medical treatment. The second annual report proudly noted that the hospital had already provided "no inconsiderable opportunities for practical instruction" to Woman's Medical College students, as well as to student nurses.[45]

Following the Civil War, leading women physicians continued to pursue a dual strategy. They maintained and strengthened their separate woman's medical sphere, all the while advocating their ultimate goal—expanded opportunities for women in the male medical establishment.

As Elizabeth Blackwell explained, it was with mixed feelings that she and Emily decided to open a medical college for women in New York:

> In 1865 the trustees . . . applied to the Legislature for a charter conferring college powers upon [the infirmary].
> . . . We took this step, however, with hesitation, for our feeling was adverse to the formation of an entirely separate school for women. The first women physicians connected with the infirmary, having all been educated in the ordinary medical schools, felt very strongly the advantage of admission to the large organized system of public instruction already existing for men. . . . Finding, however, after consultation with the different New York schools, that such arrangements could not at present be made, the trustees . . . opened a subscription for a college fund.[46]

The Woman's Medical College of the New York Infirmary, like its sister institution in Philadelphia, was an innovator from the start. A course in

[Women physicians] represent not only a profession, but a cause; the noble and holy cause of woman's advancement. —Dr. Henry Hartshorne

Higher education for women produces monstrous brains and puny bodies, abnormally active cerebration and abnormally weak digestion, flowing thought and constipated bowels. —Dr. E. H. Clarke

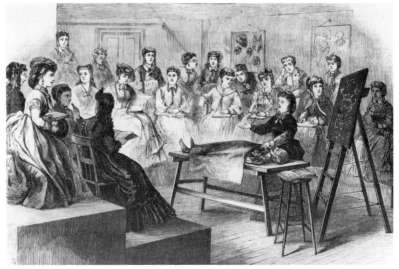

Portrait of the anatomy lecture room at the Woman's Medical College of the New York Infirmary, Frank Leslie's Illustrated Newspaper, *April 16, 1870.* New York Infirmary/Beekman Downtown Hospital.

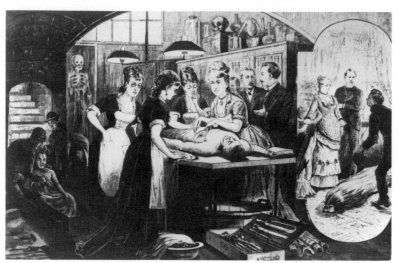

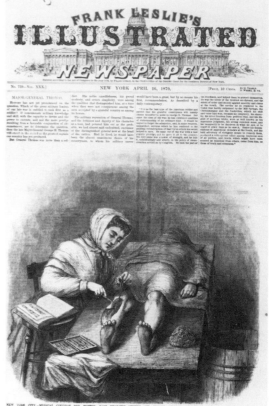

Caricature of students at the Woman's Medical College of the New York Infirmary "finding out with the aid of a lancet the peculiarities of the masculine heart," Frank Leslie's Illustrated Newspaper, *April 16, 1870.* New York Infirmary/Beekman Downtown Hospital.

Illustration of student dissecting at the Woman's Medical College of the New York Infirmary (1870). New York Public Library.

Although women make the best nurses, they do not inspire confidence as doctors since their judgement varies from month to month.
— Dr. Horatio Storer

hygiene was established, an independent examining board was founded, and the college course was lengthened from three to four years.

In 1869, Ann Preston, now dean of the hardy Woman's Medical College of Pennsylvania, at last made some headway in her long campaign for equal access to the male-controlled teaching clinics. On January 2 of that year, a major breakthrough occurred when women students were invited to attend lectures at Philadelphia Hospital's Blockley Almshouse. Dr. Alfred Stillé, a distinguished clinician and a future president of the American Medical Association, addressed the class:

> Ladies and Gentlemen, I have pleasure in welcoming you today. It is the first time . . . that I have had the opportunity of addressing women among the audience of my pupils. We are sometimes shocked at what is novel, simply because it gives us an unaccustomed impression, but in the present instance I must say that, as far as I am personally concerned, I not only have no objection to seeing ladies among a medical audience, but . . . I welcome them.[47]

Other city hospitals followed Blockley's lead, although not always with the same dignity. In the fall, Pennsylvania Hospital indicated that the students

SEND US A LADY PHYSICIAN

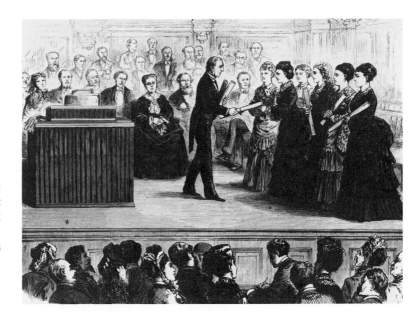

Commencement exercises of the Woman's Medical College of the New York Infirmary, at Steinway Hall, Frank Leslie's Illustrated Newspaper, *April 16, 1870.* New York Infirmary/Beekman Downtown Hospital.

of the Woman's Medical College might purchase tickets and attend hospital lectures.

Ann Preston and thirty of her students duly proceeded to the lecture hall, where they met with a less than cordial reception. One of those students, Elizabeth Keller, later senior surgeon at the New England Hospital for Women and Children, described that fateful day: "We entered in a body, amidst jeerings, groaning, whistlings, and stamping of feet by the men students. . . . On leaving the hospital, we were actually stoned by those so-called gentlemen."[48] The Philadelphia *Evening Bulletin* provided an equally vivid account of the whole affair:

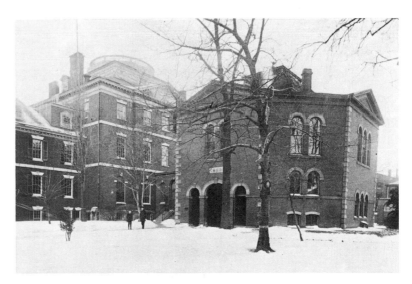

The Pennsylvania Hospital, founded in 1868. The Pennsylvania Hospital.

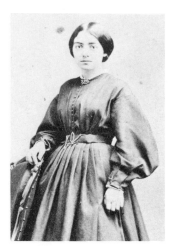

Dr. Mary Putnam Jacobi, 1842–1906 (1865). The Schlesinger Library, Radcliffe College.

A woman can love and respect her family just as much if not more when she feels that she is supporting herself and adding to their comfort and happiness.

—Dr. Georgiana Glenn

SEND US A LADY PHYSICIAN

The students of the male colleges . . . turned out several hundred strong. . . .

Ranging themselves in line, these gallant gentlemen assailed the young ladies . . . with insolent and offensive language, and then followed them into the street, where the whole gang . . . joined in insulting them. . . .

During the last hour missiles of paper, tinfoil, tobacco-quids, etc., were thrown upon the ladies, while some of these men defiled the dresses of the ladies near them with tobacco-juice.[49]

Replying in the Philadelphia newspapers to a published protest against co-education at clinical lectures, Ann Preston agreed that in operations involving "embarrassing exposure of the person,"[50] it was proper for men to treat men and women to treat women. She added, however, "we maintain that wherever it is proper to introduce women as patients, there also it is but just and in accordance with the instincts of the truest womanhood for women to appear as physicians and students."[51] To their credit, the managers of the Pennsylvania Hospital stood firm in their support of the women's right to attend the mixed lectures.

Although opportunities for clinical training for female medical students were expanding, no similar expansion in postgraduate internships occurred. Thwarted in their attempts to intern in America's more advanced hospitals, many women physicians sought clinical experience in Europe. Ironically, their choice, though forced by discrimination at home, afforded women physicians superior training at the scientifically advanced European institutions. One of the best and brightest nineteenth-century women physicians was a product of just such an education.

Mary Putnam Jacobi had decided on a career in science as a young girl. The eldest of eleven children born to publisher George Palmer Putnam and wife Victorine Haven Putnam, she received her elementary education from her mother at home. At the age of twenty, she enrolled in the New York College of Pharmacy, graduating in 1863. Although her announced plan to attend the Woman's Medical College of Pennsylvania met with parental concern, she matriculated in 1863, at the age of twenty-one. A few days after her arrival in Philadelphia, Jacobi received a letter of fatherly advice: "Now Minnie, you know very well that I am proud of your abilities [but] . . . Be a lady from the dotting of your i's to the color of your ribbons—and if you must be a doctor and a philosopher, be an attractive and agreeable one."[52]

Because of her previous experience and considerably scholarly talents, Jacobi was graduated from the Woman's Medical College of Pennsylvania in one short year. After completing an internship at the New England Hospital for Women and Children under Marie Zakrzewska and Lucy Sewall, she determined that the kind of scientific educaton she required was available only in Europe. In 1866, she set sail for Paris, where at the world-famous Ecole de Médecine she hoped to supplement the training she had received in America. Settling in a Paris pension arranged by Elizabeth Blackwell, Jacobi wrote to her mother explaining her reasons for seeking European training: "I . . . have already sufficient terror of . . . New York, with its very slack interest in medical science or progress, its deficient libraries, badly organized schools and hospitals, etc. I am doing my best . . . to make headway against these adverse influences. . . ."[53]

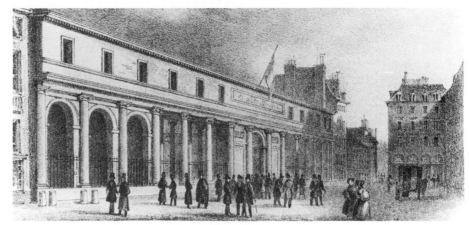

The Ecole de Médecine in Paris (c. 1829). NLM.

Even as Jacobi was lobbying for formal admission into the Ecole de Médecine, she was making ambitious plans for her return to America, including "the creation of a scientific spirit (which at present does not exist) among women medical students," "entrée into the New York Academy of Medicine," and "pursuit of numerous important problems in experimental therapeutics."

This dedication to scientific excellence would place Jacobi in a pivotal position in the American women's medical movement. She, more than any other nineteenth-century woman physician, insisted that human compassion and pure science were *equally* essential to the practice of good medicine. Through her writings and by her example, Jacobi sought to raise scientific standards in both classroom and clinical training for women physicians. Jacobi's personal goals, outlined in a letter to her mother dated 1870, revealed her generous spirit and seriousness of purpose:

1st: To honestly earn my living . . .
2nd: To pay my debts . . .
3rd: To educate the younger children . . .
4th: To buy you silk dresses . . .
5th: To accumulate a medical library . . . and to secure its employent for all medical students, especially women . . .
6th: To have a fund by which I can pay for the services of a reader during the last ten years of my life, when I shall most probably be blind.[54]

After two years of attending clinics, lectures, and laboratories, at the Ecole de Médecine, Jacobi realized her dream of being formally accepted as a student. This was the first of many successes she would have in gaining access to medical institutions previously closed to women. A brilliant scientific scholar, Jacobi passed her examinations with high honors and received the coveted Bronze Medal for her thesis. The *New York Evening Post* proudly published an account of the young American's achievements:

In Paris, on the 24th of July, Miss Putnam . . . submitted her thesis of doctor before the medical faculty. The examiners . . . addressed her flattering compli-

The danger comes from the faulty system of female education, the decay of home life, and the unwillingness of our girls to become mothers.
—Dr. William Goodell

I fear hopeless insanity, brought on by over brain work at school. Four of my cases of very bad nervous exhaustion were graduates of our best known female colleges. —Dr. William Goodell

WILL THERE BE A MONUMENT?

97

ments on the remarkable manner in which she treated the subject . . . at the same time bestowing upon the fair graduate the highest mark that is ever given—that of "perfectly satisfactory."[55]

Writing to her mother of the graduation, Jacobi expressed regret at her father's absence. "I was sorry that Father could not be in Paris in time; I think he would have been amused to see me wearing the robe . . . suiting a woman as well as a man."[56]

In 1871, Jacobi returned to America to teach at the Woman's Medical College of the New York Infirmary, which Emily Blackwell had been running since her sister's departure for England in 1869. For over a decade Jacobi taught challenging courses in Materia Medica at the college, working toward her early goal of instilling a scientific spirit in women medical students.

In July of 1873 she married Dr. Abraham Jacobi, a German revolutionary who had emigrated to the United States. When they met in New York, Abraham Jacobi was well established as one of the leading pediatricians in the country. In the course of their long marriage she bore him three children, of which only one, a daughter, survived to adulthood. In her private life as in her public life, Jacobi set an example for other women: it was possible to have a career and a family too.

Mary Putnam Jacobi, like most leaders of the nineteenth-century women's medical movement, believed the progress of women doctors was intimately entwined with the progress of all women. She was instrumental in establishing the Working Women's Society (after 1890 the New York Consumers' League) and worked for suffrage in New York, publishing *Common Sense as Applied to Women Suffrage* in 1894.

In her active participation in the general women's rights struggle, Jacobi was not alone.

As early as 1850, Harriot Hunt addressed the Woman's Rights Convention in Worcester, Massachusetts. In her autobiography, Hunt recalled her initial reaction to the planned convention and the public's misunderstanding of its purposes:

This call for a convention was such a fulfillment of unuttered hopes. . . .

On my arrival in Boston, I was assailed with such questions as these: "Then you wish to be a man? . . . So you are going to take man's place?" . . . I was astonished at the . . . misconception. The idea of the subjugation of man, instead of the elevation of woman, appeared to have taken possession of the public mind.[57]

In 1852, Ann Preston inspired participants at the Woman's Rights Convention in West Chester, Pennsylvania, explaining, "There is, at this time, a vast amount of unhappiness among women for want of free outlets to their powers; . . . thousands are yearning for fuller development, and a wider field of usefulness." Preston went on to point out, "Even for the same services, woman generally receives less than man. The whole tendency of our customs, habits and teaching is to make her *dependent*—dependent in outward circumstances, dependent in spirit."[58]

Marie Zakrzewska did her part as well. An enthusiastic participant in the

SEND US A LADY PHYSICIAN

suffrage movement, she helped found the influential New England Woman's Club.

The larger women's movement repaid the support of women physicians in kind, often advocating the placement of women doctors in public positions of leadership—as heads of women's departments in hospitals and prisons, and as school physicians. Still there were matters that required the attention of separate organizations of women doctors.

In 1872, Mary Putnam Jacobi organized the Association for the Advancement of the Medical Education for Women, serving as president from 1874–1903. In addition to raising the standards of medical education for women, this group, like the alumnae associations of the Woman's Medical College of the New York Infirmary and the Woman's Medical College of Pennsylvania, served as a connecting link among women doctors throughout the country. In an 1883 commencement address to graduates of the Woman's Medical College of the New York Infirmary, Jacobi urged a new crop of women graduates to organize against the opposition:

> You must combine to remove the difficulties which stand in your way as a class. . . . The habitual exclusion of women from fit opportunities . . . engenders a habitually low tone of confidence in their abilities, which constantly interferes to prevent any given woman from demonstrating her abilities. We have not yet reached the time when it will be considered as natural for a family to employ a woman physician as a man; or where the profession of medicine will be evenly distributed between men and women. . . . To bring about this state . . . requires much effort, individual and collective, persistent, patient, far-sighted, indomitable.[59]

Throughout her career, Mary Putnam Jacobi was a favorite spokesperson for the nineteenth-century women's medical movement. As the following excerpts from the same address show, she was able simultaneously to inspire loyalty to the women's medical institutions and to encourage progress toward the movement's goals of equality in the larger medical establishment:

> You should be continually exerting yourselves to increase the education advantages of the school of which you are an alumnae and also to extend the opportunities for undergraduate education elsewhere. . . .
> The . . . hostility to women physicians, which had marked every step in . . . our thirty years' war . . . has much abated. . . . The habit of consulting women practitioners has been established . . . but the effort to exclude women from the full privileges of the profession still continues. . . .
> To overcome all this opposition, it is necessary . . . to make persistent application . . . to engage . . . without aid of their stimulus, in the same work in which they are engaged. . . . The task is difficult, but it is by no means impossible.[60]

Persistent application on the part of Mary Putnam Jacobi and hundreds of medical women and their supporters was rewarded by a succession of victories. By the century's end, none could fail to notice how far they had come.

Urged on by their professional associations, women physicians were publishing. In 1895, Dr. Clara Marshall at the Woman's Medical College of

Public examinations, recitations, exhibitions, and commencements . . . teach [girls] how to face an audience but not how to make a home.
—Dr. William Goodell

I see woman gathering up her soul and personality and claiming them as her own against all the odds and the world. —Mary S. Howell

The girl of the future will select her own avocation and take her own training for it.
—Ruth C. D. Havens

WILL THERE BE A MONUMENT?

No. 1. (*continued.*)

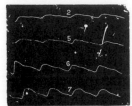

Jan. 2d. Pulse 100. 5th day after menses.

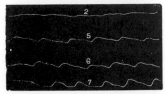

Jan. 7th. 10th day after menses.

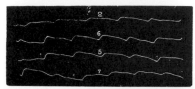

Jan. 11th. 14th day after menses.

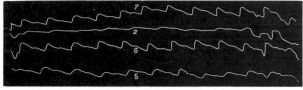

Jan. 14th 9 days before menses.

*Sphygmographic charts used to illustrate Dr. Mary
Putnam Jacobi's prizewinning essay, "The Question of
Rest for Women during Menstruation," 1876.* Ruth J.
Abram Collection.

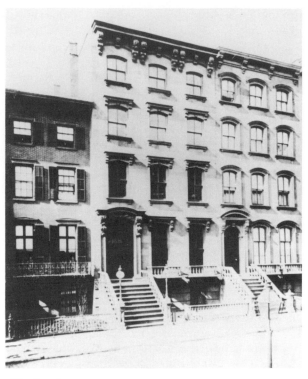

*The first home of the New York Academy of Medicine,
12 West Thirty-first Street, 1874–90.* NYAM.

Pennsylvania, proudly published a list of the publications of the school's graduates. They numbered over five hundred. Jacobi herself was responsible for over one hundred, and one of them, an essay entitled "The Question of Rest for Women during Menstruation," had won the coveted Boylston Prize from Harvard for the best essay in medicine. As the judging was blind, the essayists' names being withheld from the panel, they had not realized that the prizewinner was a woman. Jacobi's essay, which now carried the weight of the distinguished award, argued persuasively against the idea that menstruating women required rest—an argument frequently used to deny women positions of responsibility.

State and local medical societies routinely accepted women. Even the national American Medical Association, which would not elect a woman to membership until 1915, seated Dr. Sarah Hackett Stevenson at the 1876 convention as the duly elected delegate from Chicago's Medical Society. In New York, Mary Putnam Jacobi opened the doors for women with her election to membership in a succession of prestigious medical societies, including the New York Academy of Medicine, the New York Pathological Society, and the Therapeutical Society.

One of the most exciting developments of all was the beginning of acceptance of women as physicians and teachers in the male-run hospitals and schools. Again Dr. Jacobi was in the lead. In 1873, she helped establish a children's dispensary at Mt. Sinai Hospital in New York, the precursor to its pediatrics ward. In 1882, she accepted a post on the faculty of the New York Post-Graduate Medical School. In 1893, Dr. Jacobi was appointed visiting physician at St. Mark's Hospital.

In 1881, determined to break the remaining barriers to medical education for women, a committee including Marie Zakrzewska and Emily Blackwell raised fifty thousand dollars, which was offered to Harvard on the condition that women students be accepted. Although Harvard declined the offer, the strategy succeeded at Johns Hopkins a decade later.

In 1893, with the famed Dr. William Osler as its physician-in-chief, Johns Hopkins University opened its medical school, inviting women to apply.

Writing of the opening, Boston Cardinal James Gibbons cited the older argument for women in medicine, saying that "The alleviation of suffering, for women of all classes, which would result from the presence among us of an adequate number of well-trained female physicians, cannot but be evident to all; but I wish to emphasize . . . the moral influence of such a body; . . . there could be no more potent factor in the moral regeneration of society."[61]

Dr. Mary Putnam Jacobi wrote too, again delicately balancing the dual

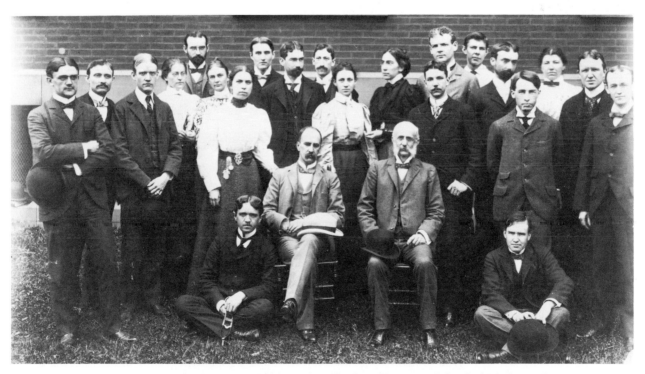

Medical school class, Johns Hopkins University School of Medicine (late 1890s). NLM.

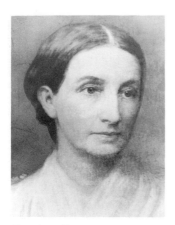

Dr. Ann Preston.
ASCWM, MCP.

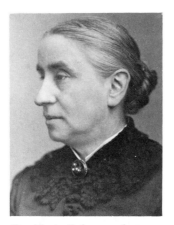

*Dr. Marie Zakrezewska
(1880s).* Robinson Family
Collection.

strategies. "It is essential," she began, "to the efficiency and the reputation of women's colleges that women should not be educated exclusively in them."[62]

Dr. William Osler promised that Johns Hopkins would "prove a new departure in medical education in this country, exacting a higher standard and more prolonged term of study."[63]

Johns Hopkins's commitment to women's medical education prompted others to follow. Cornell University's decision to admit women to its medical school in 1898 underscored the point that coeducation was the wave of the future.

In June 1899, the trustees of the Woman's Medical College of the New York Infirmary closed the school. In the school's last announcement, Dr. Emily Blackwell explained the reasons. "The friends who established, and have supported, the Infirmary and its College have always regarded co-education at the final stage in the medical education of women." But as "medical education may hereafter be obtained by women in New York in the same classes, under the same faculty, and with the same clinical opportunities as men,"[64] it seemed to Blackwell and the trustees that their work was done. This view was widely shared. Only two of the nineteen women's medical colleges founded in the nineteenth century continued into the twentieth.

Traveling in Europe in 1881 for a well-deserved rest, Marie Zakrzewska gazed at the busts of famous men adorning the halls of Westminster Abbey and wondered,

> Will there ever be a monument to the first woman physician because she was the leader of the movement; because she had the energy, will and talent, . . . and because she is a landmark of the era marked by women's freeing themselves from the bondage of prejudice and from the belief that they are the lower being when compared with men?
>
> . . . We need such landmarks of civilization . . . because the now-living, as well as those who will live long afterward, need encouragement. . . . The person who is covered by a monument is of no consequence, but the fact that a "woman" can work and make an impression upon civilization needs to be known and to be remembered.[65]

On April 18, 1871, fifty-eight-year-old Ann Preston died at home. "Ann Preston was the College and the College was Ann Preston," commented a colleague.[66] Dr. Eliza Judson said of Ann Preston, "To the cause of woman, her work and example were invaluable. . . . Her life was an unanswerable argument against those who would exclude women from the medical profession."[67]

Harriot Hunt died four years later and was laid to rest under a statue of Hygeia, goddess of health, which she had commissioned from black sculptor Edmonia Lewis.

As these two great figures left the stage, new advocates stepped up to join the remaining older pioneers, women and men alike, to carry on.

On May 12, 1902, after an illness of three years, Marie Zakrzewska died. Her farewell letter was read to the mourners.

> I do not think that my name . . . will be remembered. Yet the idea for which I have worked . . . must live and spread. . . .

I desire no hereafter. I was born; I lived; I used my life to the best of my ability for the uplifting of my fellow creatures; and I enjoyed it daily in a thousand ways.[68]

Mary Putnam Jacobi died on June 6, 1906, but not before writing "Early Symptoms of the Meningeal Tumor Compressing the Cerebellum," a detailed description of the affliction that killed her. In her life, Jacobi realized the dream she described at the age of ten in a letter to her grandmother:

Vague longings beset me. I imagine great things and glorious deeds; but Ah! the vision passes like a fleeting dream and the muddy reality is left behind. I would be great. I would do deeds, so that after I had passed into that world, that region beyond the grave, I should be spoken of with affection so that I should live again in the hearts of those I have left behind me.[69]

Emily and Elizabeth Blackwell died a few months apart in 1910. Theirs had been lives of triumphs over considerable odds. Even their ultimate dream of coeducation at the better medical schools had been realized. There were over seven thousand women physicians practicing throughout the United States and beyond. The Blackwells could remember a time when there were none.

In 1893, Dr. Anna Fullerton, physician in charge of the Woman's Hospital, Philadelphia, paid tribute to the early pioneers:

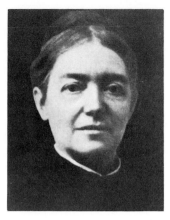

Dr. Mary Putnam Jacobi (1880s). Ruth J. Abram Collection.

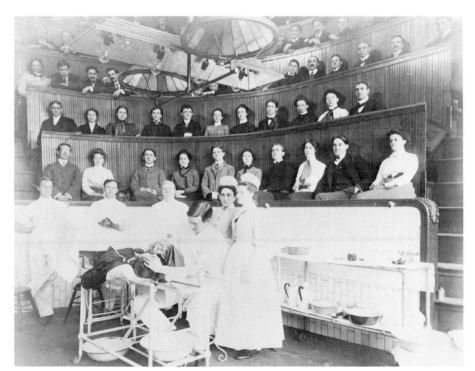

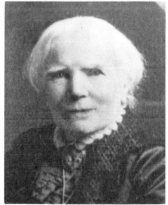

Dr. Elizabeth Blackwell in her seventies (c. 1895). New York Infirmary/Beekman Downtown Hospital.

Surgical clinic, Cornell Medical College (1890s). Medical Archives, New York Hospital, Cornell Medical Center.

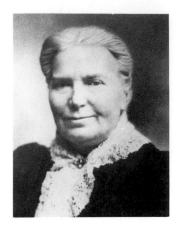

Dr. Emily Blackwell, 1826–1910. New York Infirmary/Beekman Downtown Hospital.

In the pursuit of medicine, the advancement of woman's cause . . . [these] pioneers—both men and women—suffered chill and utter loneliness in the performance of a duty upon which the world looked coldly. For us they were misunderstood and despised and calumniated; for us they went on the forlorn hope of truth in a service of peril to their own happiness, and we cannot afford to forget them.[70]

NOTES

1. Harriot Hunt, *Glances and Glimpses; or Fifty Years of Social, Including Twenty Years Professional Life* [*sic*] (Boston: John P. Jewett and Company, 1856), 152.
2. Elizabeth Blackwell, *Pioneer Work in Opening the Medical Profession to Women: Autobiographical Sketches by Dr. Elizabeth Blackwell* (New York: Schocken, 1977 reprint of 1895 edition), 27–29.
3. Blackwell, *Opening the Medical Profession to Women*, 59–60.
4. Ibid., 31.
5. Ibid., 35.
6. Ibid., 66.
7. Hunt, *Glances and Glimpses*, 267.
8. Ibid., 270.
9. Blackwell, *Opening the Medical Profession to Women*, 72.
10. Ibid., 80.
11. Edward T. James, ed., *Notable American Women* (Cambridge, MA: The Belknap Press of Harvard University Press, 1971), 165.
12. Dr. Joseph Longshore, "Valedictory Address Delivered Before the Class at the First Annual Commencement of the Female Medical College of Pennsylvania," December 30, 1851; Archives and Special Collections on Women in Medicine, Medical College of Pennsylvania. (The college opened as the Female Medical College of Pennsylvania; in 1867, the name was changed to the Woman's Medical College of Pennsylvania; and in 1970, the named was changed to the Medical College of Pennsylvania.)
13. Blackwell, *Opening the Medical Profession to Women*, 190–96.
14. Ibid., 197–98.
15. Dr. Elizabeth Blackwell to Dr. Gertrude Walker (Recording Secretary, Alumnae Association) at the time of the Fiftieth Anniversary of the founding of the Woman's Medical College of Pennsylvania, April 21, 1900; Archives and Special Collection on Women in Medicine, Medical College of Pennsylvania.
16. Ann Preston to an unnamed man, December 19, 1852, Chester County (Pennsylvania) Historical Society.
17. Blackwell, *Opening the Medical Profession to Women*, app. III, 261–64.
18. Agnes C. Vietor, M.D., F.A.C.S., ed., *A Woman's Quest: The Life of Marie E. Zakrzewska, M.D.* (New York and London: D. Appleton and Company, 1924), 84–85.
19. Ibid., 108–10.
20. Blackwell, *Opening the Medical Profession to Women*, 201.
21. Vietor, *A Woman's Quest*, 142.
22. Ibid., 179–80.
23. The members of the Blackwell family living with Elizabeth at this time included her mother, Hannah (Lane) Blackwell (an abolitionist); her brother Samuel Blackwell and his wife, Antoinette Brown Blackwell (the first American woman minister); and her brother Henry Blackwell (an abolitionist) and his wife, Lucy Stone (an antislavery and women's rights leader).
24. Vietor, *A Woman's Quest*, 192.

25. Blackwell, *Opening the Medical Profession to Women,* 209.
26. Vietor, *A Woman's Quest,* 212.
27. Ibid., 210–11.
28. Blackwell, *Opening the Medical Profession to Women,* 209.
29. Vietor, *A Woman's Quest,* 219.
30. Ibid., 219.
31. Ibid., 213–14.
32. Blackwell, *Opening the Medical Profession to Women,* 227.
33. Ibid., 227–28.
34. Ann Preston, *Introductory Lectures and Valedictory Addresses,* 1855, 8; Archives and Special Collections on Women in Medicine, Medical College of Pennsylvania.
35. Ibid.
36. Gulielma Fell Alsop, M.D., *History of the Woman's Medical College, Philadelphia, Pennsylvania, 1850–1950* (Philadelphia, London, and Montreal: J. B. Lippincott Company, 1950), 61.
37. Ibid., 63.
38. Vietor, *A Woman's Quest,* 268–69.
39. Ibid., 251.
40. Ibid.
41. Blackwell, *Opening the Medical Profession to Women,* 234.
42. Ibid., 295.
43. Ibid., 192.
44. Alsop, *History of the Woman's Medical College,* 48.
45. "Charter and By-Laws of the Woman's Hospital of Philadelphia, with the First Annual Report of the Board of Managers," January 1862, 12; and "Second Annual Report of the Board of Managers of the Woman's Hospital of Philadelphia," January 1863, 6: Archives and Special Collections on Women in Medicine, Medical College of Pennsylvania.
46. Blackwell, *Opening the Medical Profession to Women,* 238.
47. Eliza E. Judson, "Address in Memory of Ann Preston, M.D.," March 11, 1873; Archives and Special Collections on Women in Medicine, Medical College of Pennsylvania.
48. Woman's Medical College of Pennsylvania: Transactions of the Alumnae Association, 1906, 61.
49. Alsop, *History of the Woman's Medical College,* 54–55.
50. Ibid., 56.
51. Ibid., 57.
52. Ruth Putnam, ed. *Life and Letters, Mary Putnam Jacobi* (New York and London; G. P. Putnam's Sons, 1925); 67.
53. *Life and Letters of Mary Putnam Jacobi,* 233.
54. Ibid., 234–235.
55. Ibid., 289.
56. Ibid., 287.
57. Hunt, *Glances and Glimpses,* 251–56.
58. Ann Preston, address adopted by the Woman's Rights Convention held in West Chester, Pennsylvania, June 2–3, 1852; Archives and Special Collections on Women in Medicine, Medical College of Pennsylvania.
59. The Women's Medical Association of New York City, eds., *Mary Putnam Jacobi, M.D.: A Pathfinder in Medicine* (New York and London: G. P. Putnam's Sons, 1925), 397.
60. Ibid., 400.
61. "The Opening of the Johns Hopkins Medical School to Women," February 1891; The Schlesinger Library, Radcliffe College.

62. Ibid.

63. Ibid.

64. Final catalogue and announcement, the Woman's Medical College of the New York Infirmary for Women and Children, June 1899; New York Infirmary/Beekman Downtown Hospital Archives, New York.

65. Vietor, *A Woman's Quest,* 404–5.

66. Alsop, *History of the Woman's Medical College,* 26.

67. Eliza E. Judson, "Address in Memory of Ann Preston, M.D.," March 11, 1873; Archives and Special Collections on Women in Medicine, Medical College of Pennsylvania.

68. Vietor, *A Woman's Quest,* 475–77.

69. The Women's Medical Association of New York City, *Mary Putnam Jacobi, M.D.,* xxx.

70. Ann M. Fullerton, M.D., "Woman in Medicine: Her Duties and Responsibilities," an address to the graduates of the Woman's Medical College of Pennsylvania, May 3, 1893; Archives and Special Collections on Women in Medicine, Medical College of Pennsylvania.

Co-Laborers in the Work of the Lord

Nineteenth-Century Black Women Physicians

DARLENE CLARK HINE

THE Afro-American woman physician of the late nineteenth and early twentieth centuries remains an enigma. Today only scattered bits and pieces of evidence—an occasional biographical sketch, a random name in an old medical school catalogue—attest to the existence of this first generation of black women doctors. In spite of this negligible evidence, we know that in the quarter century after the demise of slavery and during the height of racial segregation and discrimination, 115 black women had become physicians in the United States.[1]

An examination of their lives and experiences will illuminate the conditions in and the transformations of the American medical profession in the last half of the nineteenth and the first quarter of the twentieth century. If white women, black men, and poor whites, as many scholars argue, were outsiders in medicine, then black women, belonging as they did to two subordinate groups, surely inhabited the most distant perimeters of the profession.[2] Yet

The author wishes to thank Professor William C. Hine of South Carolina State College for his thoughtful and helpful comments on this essay. A special word of thanks is owed to Ms. Cynthia Fitz Simmons for her research and typing assistance and to Ms. Ruth Abram and Ms. Margaret Jerrido, for their encouragement and support.

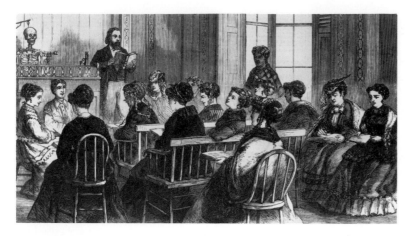

Rebecca Cole in the General lecture room, Woman's Medical College of the New York Infirmary (1870). NYAM.

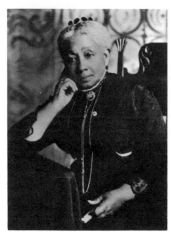

Dr. Susan Smith McKinney Steward, 1848–1919 (1890s). ASCWM, MCP.

it is precisely because of this dual—sexual and racial—marginality that any examination of their lives and careers bears the possibility of shedding new light on many conventional interpretations in American medical history.

To be sure, the history of black women physicians is one worthy of study in its own right. From an analysis of factors ranging from family background, to medical education, to medical practice, to social status, to marriage, to Victorian sex role definitions, a portrait of one of the earliest and most significant groups of black professional women emerges. Finally, insights gleaned from looking at the early black women doctors will further the reconstruction of a more inclusive and, perhaps, more accurate picture of the opportunities and restrictions that all women and black male physicians encountered in pursuit of medical careers.

In 1864, one year before the Civil War ended and fifteen years after Elizabeth Blackwell became the first American woman medical graduate, the first black woman graduate, Rebecca Lee, received an M.D. degree from the New England Female Medical College in Boston. Three years later, one year before the ratification of the Fourteenth Amendment to the United States Constitution, the second black American woman physician, Rebecca J. Cole (1846–1922), was graduated from the Woman's Medical College of Pennsylvania. They were followed by Susan Smith McKinney Steward (1848–1919), who completed her studies at New York Medical College for Women in 1870.[3] Lee, Cole, and Steward signaled the emergence of black women in the medical profession.

During this era, white women, like blacks in general, challenged traditional subservient roles and demanded improved educational opportunities and greater individual autonomy. Medical school matriculation statistics reflect the efforts and desires of many middle-class white and black women to expand restrictive private spheres to encompass areas outside of the home. The late nineteenth century witnessed a dramatic increase of women doctors in America. Their numbers rose from a mere 200 or fewer in 1860 to 2,423 in 1880 and to more than 7,000 by 1900. During this period nineteen medical schools for women were founded, although by 1895 eleven had disbanded.[4] By the 1920s the United States Census listed only 65 black women as actually practicing phy-

SEND US A LADY PHYSICIAN

sicians. Not surprisingly, black male physicians far outnumbered their female counterparts. In 1890 there were 909 black physicians; by 1920 the number had jumped to 3,885.[5]

The increase in the numbers of black physicians was due largely to the existence of several medical schools founded for blacks in the post-Reconstruction South. At one time seven such institutions flourished. (See p. 118.) Four of the seven schools were considered by black and white observers to be adequate. According to one contemporary black male physician, M. Vandehurst Lynk, the big four—Howard University School of Medicine in Washington, D.C.; Meharry Medical School in Nashville, Tennessee; Leonard Medical School of Shaw University in Raleigh, North Carolina; and Flint Medical College (originally known as the Medical Department of New Orleans University) in New Orleans, Louisiana—labored to keep up with quickly evolving medical standards. They "not only extended the instruction over four years, but have increased the number of subjects to be taught and have better equipped facilities," Lynk wrote in 1893.[6] By 1914, however, of the approved medical schools only Howard and Meharry remained open. These two institutions played the most significant role in the education of black women physicians.

The Howard University Medical School, chartered in 1868 and supported by the United States government as an institution to train blacks for the medical profession, actually had more white students than black during the early years. The founders of the Howard Medical School had all been officers in the Union Army, including Dr. Alexander T. Augusta, the only black on the original faculty. The first woman faculty member was Isabel C. Barrows, who was graduated from the Woman's Medical College in New York City and who studied opthalmology in Vienna. She lectured on this subject at Howard in 1872 and 1873.[7]

By 1900 Howard University had graduated 552 physicians, 35 of whom, or 5 percent of the total, were women. Only 25 of the 35 women, however, were black. The first 2 women to be graduated from the medical school, Mary D. Spackman (1872) and Mary A. Parsons (1874), were white.[8]

Howard's gender-blind policy sparked outright hostility and retaliation from some medical colleges. In 1873, the school's Medical Alumni Association denounced discrimination against women "as being unmanly and unworthy of the [medical] profession," and declared, "we accord to all persons the same rights and immunities that we demand for ourselves."[9] Four years later, however, the Association of American Medical Colleges, spurred by objections of the Jefferson Medical College of Philadelphia faculty, refused to seat the Howard delegation at its annual convention, in part because the Howard Medical School permitted men and women to be taught in the same classes.[10]

Meharry Medical College in Nashville, Tennessee, actually graduated the largest number of black women physicians (thirty-nine by 1920). Beginning in 1876 as the medical department of Central Tennessee College, Meharry was the first medical school in the South to provide for the education of black physicians. In light of the fact that the majority of blacks still resided in the eleven southern states of the old Confederacy, where racial segregation and exclusionism prevailed, Meharry's location made it the logical place for the majority of black women to pursue a medical education. In 1893, seventeen years after its opening, Meharry graduated its first black women physicians, Annie D. Gregg and Georgia Esther Lee Patton. Three black women had reached junior class status in 1882 but for reasons unknown they were never graduated.[11] Meharry had a penchant for hiring its own graduates. The first woman to teach at Meharry and the first to attain a position of leadership there was Josie E. Wells, a member of the class of 1904. Wells had received prior training as a nurse. Specializing in diseases of women and children, Wells gave freely of her time and resources. She dispensed free medicine and treatment to poor blacks in Nashville two afternoons a week. As superintendent of Hubbard Hospital, the teaching facility associated with Meharry, Wells executed her duties with skill. A black male colleague wrote of her, "She was really a remarkable woman, and under a more favorable environment might have risen to fame."[12]

By the turn of the century the Woman's Medical College of Pennsylvania, established in 1850 as the first regular medical school for females, had graduated approximately a dozen black women physicians. The Woman's Medical College blazed a new trail of providing medical training to women of every race, creed, and national origin. Indeed, all of the women's medical colleges, which in most instances were founded as temporary expediencies, enabled women to escape social ostracism, subtle discrimination, and overt hostility throughout their training in a male-dominated profession. Still, integration with male medical schools remained the guiding aspiration of most women in the medical profession. Unfortunately, the trend toward coeducation in the 1870s did not signal much change in the percentage of black female physicians. Only one or two ever attended the integrated coeducational institutions.[13]

Among the early black women graduates of the Woman's Medical College were Rebecca J. Cole (1867), Caroline Still Wiley Anderson (1878), Verina Morton Jones (1888), Halle Tanner Dillon Johnson (1891), Lucy Hughes Brown (1894), Alice Woodby McKane (1894), Matilda Arabella Evans (1897), and Eliza Anna Grier (1897). Of this group a large proportion became pioneers in establishing, simultaneously, a female and a black presence in the medical profession in several southern states. Three of the early black women graduates from the Woman's Medical College—Johnson, Jones, and Brown— became the first of their sex to practice medicine in Alabama, Mississippi, and South Carolina, respectively.[14] It is open to speculation whether the successes achieved by the Woman's Medical College's black graduates attest to a high quality of education or simply underscore the advantage of a more nurturing and supportive, sex-segregated environment, in which sutdents learned from female faculty role models. Closer scrutiny suggests other factors, including family background, prior education, and social status, may have influenced their securing a medical education in the first place and subsequently their success.

That family background and prior education were important determinants of succcess in acquiring a medical education is reflected in the lives of a few of the early black women physicians, such as Caroline Still Wiley Anderson and Halle Tanner Dillon Johnson. The majority of the early black women physicians were the daughters of socially privileged or "representative" black families who, perhaps to protect them from menial labor or domestic servitude, encouraged their daughters to educate themselves. Of the few career options open to black women, teaching was the most accessible profession. Indeed, outside of the professions of teaching, medicine, and nursing, black women possessed scant opportunity for white- or pink-collar jobs as sales clerks, elevator operators, or typists. Ironically, they either entered the professions at the outset or remained mired in service occupations; there was little in between.[15]

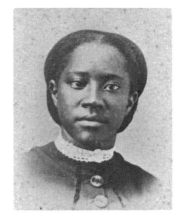

Dr. Caroline Still Wiley Anderson (1848–1919). Oberlin College Archives.

Caroline Still Wiley Anderson (1848–1919) was the daughter of William and Letitia Still of Philadelphia. Her father had achieved widespread fame as a founder of the Underground Railroad and Vigilance Committee in antebellum Philadelphia and as the author of *The Underground Railroad,* which chronicled the means and patterns of escape for runaway slaves. Anderson received her primary and secondary education at Mrs. Henry Gordon's Private School, The Friends Raspberry Alley School, and the Institute for Colored Youth. She entered Oberlin College, in 1874, the only black woman in a class of forty-six. Upon graduation she married a black classmate; after his premature death she moved to Washington, D.C., where she taught music and gave instruction in drawing and elocution at Howard University. She completed one term at the Howard University Medical School before entering, in 1876, the Woman's Medical College in Philadelphia. In 1880 she married a prominent minister and educator, Matthew Anderson.[16]

Halle Tanner Dillon Johnson, born in 1864 in Pittsburgh, was also a member of an outstanding family. She was the daughter of Bishop B. T. Tanner of the African Methodist Episcopal Church in Philadelphia.[17] Sarah Logan Fraser, a New York native, was the daughter of Bishop Logan of the Zion Methodist Episcopal Church. Like William Still, Bishop Logan had aided and harbored escaping slaves in his home, in Syracuse, New York.[18] Unlike Caroline Still Wiley Anderson and Halle Tanner Dillon Johnson, Fraser received her medical degree from the Medical School of Syracuse University. Another New Yorker, Susan Smith McKinney Steward, the seventh of ten children born to Sylvanus and Anne Springsteel Smith, was the daughter of a prosperous Brooklyn pork merchant. One of her sisters was married to the noted antislavery leader Reverend Henry Highland Garnett.[19] Among Southern black women doctors, Sarah G. Boyd Jones is a good example of a daughter of a representative black family who enjoyed a highly successful medical career. Her father, George W. Boyd, was reputed to be the wealthiest black man in Richmond. A native of Albermale County, Virginia, Sarah attended the Richmond Normal School before completing medical training in 1893 at Howard University Medical School. After graduation she returned to Richmond, where she became the first woman to pass the Virginia medical board examinations. She later founded the Richmond Hospital and Training School of Nurses, which in 1902 was renamed the Sarah G. Jones Memorial Hospital.[20]

To be sure, not all of the first generation of black women physicians belonged to illustrious and socially prominent families. They had, however, received the best undergraduate preparations then available to blacks. Some,

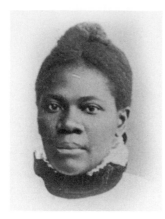

Dr. Eliza Grier, 18–?–1902 (1890s). ASCWM, MCP.

such as Eliza Anna Grier, were former slaves who worked their way through college and medical school, occasionally receiving minimal financial assistance from parents and siblings.

It took Eliza Anna Grier seven years to work and study her way through Fisk University in Nashville, Tennessee. In 1890 she wrote to the Woman's Medical College concerning her financial straits, "I have no money and no source from which to get it only as I work for every dollar." She continued, "What I want to know from you is this. How much does it take to put one through a year in your school? Is there any possible chance to do any work that would not interfere with one's studies?" Grier apparently completed the medical program by working every other year, for it took her seven years to earn the degree. She was graduated in 1897.[21]

Even those black families who for various reasons could not afford to assist their daughters financially did, nevertheless, provide much-needed moral support and encouragement. May E. Chinn, who in 1892 became the first black woman graduate of the University of Bellevue Medical Center, noted the importance of her mother's support. Interviewed at the age of eighty-one, she recalled that her father, who had been a slave, opposed her even going to college, but her mother, who "scrubbed floors and hired out as a cook," became the driving force behind her educational effort.[22]

Black women who were fortunate enough to secure medical education in spite of limited access to and segregation and gender discrimination in the schools did so only to encounter additional obstacles. For most black women the establishment of a financially and professionally rewarding medical practice proved a most formidable challenge. Racial customs and negative attitudes toward women dictated that black women physicians practice almost exclusively among blacks, and primarily with black women, for many of whom the payment of medical fees was a great hardship. Poverty usually was accompanied by superstition and fear. Consequently, the newly minted black woman doctor frequently had to expend considerable effort persuading, cajoling, and winning confidence before being allowed to treat physical illness. May E. Chinn's experiences are again illustrative of the problems encountered. She observed that one of the peculiar problems she had to overcome as late as the 1920s was the negative attitude of some black women toward her. In one instance a black woman patient wept as Chinn approached because "she felt she had been denied the privilege of having a white doctor wait on her." Not surprisingly, few black women doctors enjoyed the support of or were consulted by their white male colleagues in the communities in which they practiced. They were, however, frequently taken aback by the actions of some of their black male colleagues. According to Chinn, black male doctors could be divided into three groups, "those who acted as if I wasn't there; another who took the attitude 'what does she think she can do that I can't do?'; and the group that called themselves supporting me by sending me their night calls after midnight."[23]

It is significant that many black women who were able to establish private practices also had to found hospitals, nursing training schools, and social service agencies. These institutions became adjuncts to their medical practices and simultaneously addressed the needs of the black communities. By custom, black professionals and patients were prohibited from using or were segregated within local health care facilities. As late as 1944 one black physician remarked, "Within the past five years, I have seen colored patients quartered in a sub-basement separated from the coal-fire furnace, of a white denominational hospital, by a thin plaster board partition not extending to the ceiling." He added, "There is much credence to be placed in the constantly repeated charge that even this concession was made only because Negro patients furnished material for the training of the white surgical staff."[24]

Several black graduates of the Woman's Medical College, most notably Lucy Hughes Brown (1863–1911) and Matilda Arabella Evans (1877–1935), journeyed south to launch medical careers. Brown, a North Carolinian by birth, moved after her 1894 graduation to Charleston, South Carolina, becoming the first black woman physician in that state. In 1896 she joined a small group of eight black male physicians led by Alonzo C. McClellan and established the Hospital and Nursing Training School.

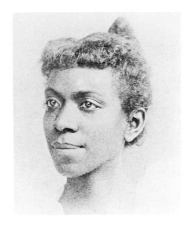

Dr. Mathilde Evans, (1869–1935). ASCWM, MCP. *caption 50.*

Matilda Arabella Evans returned after graduation to her native South Carolina, where she practiced medicine for twenty years in Columbia. Inasmuch as there were no hospital facilities open to blacks in the city, Evans initially cared for patients in her own home. Eventually, as the number of clients grew, she was able to rent a separate building with a bed capacity for thirty patients and to establish a full-scale hospital and nurses' training school. During her tenure in Columbia, she also founded the Negro Health Association of South Carolina.[25]

Black women physicians such as Rebecca J. Cole and Caroline Still Wiley Anderson skillfully combined private medical practice with community service work among white and black women. Cole worked for a time with Elizabeth and Emily Blackwell at the New York Infirmary for Women and Children as a "sanitary visitor." The Blackwells' Tenement House Service, begun in 1866, was the earliest practical program of medical social service in the country. As a sanitary visitor or "tenement physician," Cole made house calls in slum neighborhoods, teaching indigent mothers the basics of hygiene and "the preservation of health of their families." Elizabeth Blackwell described Cole as "an intelligent young coloured physician," who conducted her work "with tact and care," and thus demonstrated that the establishment of a social service department "would be a valuable addition to every hospital."[26]

After a stint in Columbia, South Carolina, during the Reconstruction, Cole returned to Philadelphia. There, with the aid of physician Charlotte Abbey, she launched a new effort on behalf of destitute women and children. In 1893 Cole and Abby founded the Woman's Directory, a medical and legal aid center. The purpose of the Woman's Directory was, according to its charter, "the prevention of feticide and infanticide and the evils connected with baby farming by rendering assistance to women in cases of approaching maternity and of desertion or abandonment of mothers and by aiding magistrates and others entrusted with police powers in preventing or punishing [such] crimes. . . ." During the latter part of her fifty-year career, Cole served as superintendent of the Government House, for children and old women, in Washington, D.C.[27]

A sister Philadelphian, Caroline Still Wiley Anderson, combined her private medical practice with the dispensary and clinic operated in conjunction with the Berean Presbyterian Church, of which her husband was the pastor. For forty years, Anderson managed the church clinic, or Berean Dispensary, as it was called, "for the benefit of women and children within the immediate neighborhood of the Church." A community activist, Anderson played a major role in establishing the first black YWCA in Philadelphia, served as treasurer of the Woman's Medical College Alumnae Association, was a member of the Women's Medical Society, and for several years occupied the position of president of the Berean Women's Christian Temperance Union. Anderson performed all of these services while maintaining her positions of assistant principal and instructor in elocution, physiology, and hygiene at the Berean Manual Training and Industrial School. In 1888 she read a paper entitled "Popliteal Aneurism," which was published in the alumnae journal of the Woman's Medical College.[28]

Given the uncertainty, costs, and emotional strain of establishing a successful private practice, it is understandable that several black women physicians initially accepted appointments as resident physicians in segregated black colleges and universities established in the South during Reconstruction. Such appointments provided small but steady stipends and much-needed experience at working in an institutional setting. Moreover, these appointments assured a degree of professional autonomy, status, and visibility and enabled the development of greater confidence.

During the 1890s and early 1900s, black women physicians Halle Tanner Dillon Johnson, Ionia R. Whipper, Verina Morton Jones, and Susan Smith McKinney Steward became resident physicians at black colleges. Not only did they minister to the health care needs of the college students and faculties, but they often taught courses and lectured on health subjects. Johnson served as a resident physician at Tuskegee Institute from 1891 to 1894. During her tenure she was responsible for the medical care of 450 students as well as for 30 officers and teachers and their families. Johnson was expected to make her own medicines, while teaching one or two classes each term. For her efforts she was paid six hundred dollars per year plus room and board; she was allowed one one-month vacation per year.[29]

In 1903, Ionia R. Whipper a member of the 1903 graduating class of Howard Medical School, succeeded Johnson and became the second black woman resident physician at Tuskegee Institute. Reflecting social change, however, Whipper was restricted to the care of female students at the institute. After leaving Tuskegee, Whipper returned to Washington, D.C., where she established a home to care for unwed, pregnant, school-age black girls. Aided by a group of seven friends, Whipper commenced this work in her home. In 1931 she purchased some property and opened the Ionia R. Whipper Home Inc. for Unwed Mothers, which had a policy of nondiscrimination as to race, religion, or residence.[30]

After completing her education at the Woman's Medical College, Verina Morton Jones accepted an appointment as a resident physician of Rust College in Holly Springs, Mississippi. Like Johnson and Whipper, Morton doubled as a teacher, giving classes to the students enrolled in the industrial school

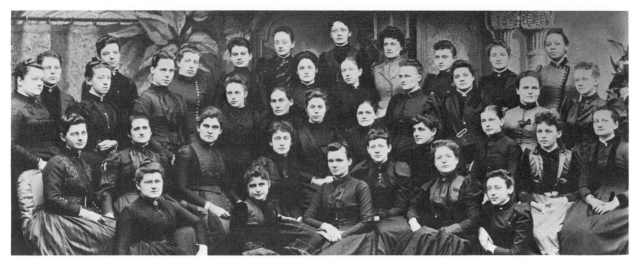

Dr. Halle Tanner Dillon Johnson with the Class of 1891, Woman's Medical College of Pennsylvania. ASCWM, MCP.

connected with the university.[31] Jones and Dillon shared another characteristic in that they both were the first women to pass their states' medical board examinations, in Alabama and Mississippi respectively.

To be sure, acquiring a medical education and establishing a practice before the turn of the century was difficult, but later generations of black women physicians were further encumbered in their pursuit of medical careers. Entrance into the medical profession became more difficult as the requirements for certification were raised. Medical graduates were increasingly expected to secure internships and residencies for specialization and to pass state medical board examinations for certification. Only a small number of the highly rated hospitals in the country accepted blacks or women for internships and residencies. Consequently, black women faced fierce competition for available slots. Most of the all-black hospitals preferred to grant internships and residencies to black men, while the few women's hospitals usually selected white women. The confluence of sexual and racial segregation strengthened the barriers blocking the aspirations and careers of black woman physicians.[32]

The experiences of Isabella Vandervall, who studied at the Woman's Medical College, reveal the difficulties involved in securing interships. Vandervall wrote in an article detailing her frustrations, "I had almost given up hope of securing an internship when one day, I saw a notice on the college bulletin board saying the Hospital for Women and Children in Syracuse, New York, wanted an interne. Here I thought was another chance. So I wrote, sent in my application, and was accepted without parley. . . . So to Syracuse I went with bag and baggage enough to last me for a year. I found the hospital; I found the superintendent. She asked me what I wanted. I told her I was Dr. Vandervall, the new interne. She simply stared and said not a word. Finally, when she came to her senses, she said to me: 'You can't come here; we can't have you here! You are colored! You will have to go back.' "[33]

As the professionalization of medicine progressed, so too increased the exclusion and ostracism of outside groups. For example, black women physicians, like their black male counterparts, chafed under the denial of membership in the leading professional organization, the American Medical Association. In response to this exclusion, black physicians met in 1895 in Atlanta, Georgia, to create the National Medical Association (NMA). From the outset, black women participated in the NMA. Although few were elected or appointed to prominent positions, they nevertheless, on occasion, held offices, attended the annual conventions, and periodically published papers in the *Journal of the National Medical Association.* For example, Georgia R. Dwelle, a graduate of Meharry who began her practice in Atlanta, Georgia, in 1906, was a vice-president of the NMA during the 1920s.[34]

In addition to their struggles with race-related problems within the medical profession, black women physicians had also to be concerned with gender-related issues. Like their white women counterparts, black women physicians remained sensitive to the prevailing social attitude that higher education and professional training threatened a woman's femininity. To be sure, black Americans, more so than white Americans, tended to tolerate women working outside the home. Economic necessity and racism so circumscribed the opportunities of black males that black women, regardless of marital status, had to contribute to the well-being of the family. Indeed, the black woman physician was frequently a much sought-after marriage partner. Many black women physicians married black ministers, fellow black physicians, or educators. Susan Smith McKinny Steward, commenting on the marriageability of black women physicians, observed, "Fortunate are the men who marry these women from an economic standpoint at least. They are blessed in a three-fold measure, in that they take unto themselves a wife, a trained nurse, and a doctor." She went on, however, to point out the necessity for the black woman physician to avoid becoming "unevenly yoked." She cautioned that "such a companion [would] prove to be a millstone hanged around her neck." Steward concluded on an optimistic note, asserting that "the medically eduated women are generally good diagnosticians in this direction also."[35]

Actually, nineteenth-century medical practice permitted the best of both worlds. Offices were frequently located in the home. Thus, marriage and career could be conducted in the same location. Aspiring black middle-class women, especially those associated with the black women's club movement and authors of the inspirational biographies of the time, vascillated in their praise of professional black women. They celebrated the accomplishments of the black women physicians and at the same time applauded the fact that these professional role models successfully fulfilled their obligations as wives and mothers. Of Steward, for example, the author of one black women's club publication declared, "She had fairly outdone her white sisters in proving that a married woman can successfully follow more than one profession without neglecting her family." In the same publication Caroline Still Wiley Anderson was hailed as a wife, mother, physician, teacher, clubwoman, and "co-laborer in the work of the Lord."[36]

Susan Smith McKinney Steward married another minister after her first husband, Reverend William C. McKinney, died. Her second husband, Reverend Theophilus G. Steward, was a former chaplain of the United States Army. An extremely successful physician, she had offices in Brooklyn and Manhattan and served on the staffs of the New York Hospital for Women, the Brooklyn Women's Homeopathic Hospital, and the Brooklyn Home for Aged Colored People. She was also a church organist and choirmaster and founded the Woman's Local Union, which was black New York's leading women's club, and the Equal Suffrage League of Brooklyn.[37]

Verina Morton Jones was also held up for commendation. She married W. A. Morton in 1890 and, after she resigned from her position as resident physician at Rust College, she and her husband established a practice in Brooklyn together, although they specialized in different areas.[38] The Brooklyn *Times* noted in 1891, "they do not interfere with each other in the least. They are a handsome young couple, intelligent and refined looking."[39] Alice Woodby McKane and her husband, Cornelius McKane, also practiced medicine as a team. In 1895 they traveled to Monrovia, Liberia, where they opened and operated the first hospital in that republic. In 1896 they returned to Savannah, Georgia, and together established the McKane Hospital for Women and Children, which was renamed Charity Hospital in the 1920s.[40]

This brief examination of black women physicians underscores the fact that much more research and discovery of additional primary source materials needs to be done before definite conclusions can be drawn concerning the impact of their work and experiences on the larger medical profession. The lives of the few women discussed reveal the depth and breadth of their struggle to overcome gender and race barriers thwarting their access to medical schools, internships, and residencies and impeding subsequent professional development. It is fair to say that in an age in which the standards of medical practice were low and the backgrounds of most physicians were wanting, these black women doctors defied, for the most part, traditional stereotypes and characterizations. This dedicated, albeit small, group of professionals was drawn, with few exceptions, from the upper echelons of black society.

Several points distinguish black women physicians, the most obvious one being that they were an integral part of the black communities in which they practiced. Moreoever, these women not only administered to the health care needs of blacks but also founded an array of related health care institutions. They established hospitals and clinics, trained nurses, taught elementary health rules to students and patients, and founded homes and service agencies for poor women and unwed girls of both races. They were self-reliant, committed, and talented women who successfully combined a multiplicity of roles as physicians, wives, mothers, daughters, and community leaders. Although they were, by any standard, elite black women, each of them employed her education and skills to the advantage of her people. It is reasonable to conclude that the convergence of the triple forces of racism, sexism, and professionalization resulted in a significant reduction in the number of black women physicians in the 1920s. It is also likely, however, that instead of entering the medical profession the aspiring, career-oriented, black women began focusing on nursing as a more viable alternative for a professionally rewarding place in the American health care system. Thus, these early black professional women played an undeniably significant role in the overall survival struggle of all black people. For their contributions, sacrifices, and services, all black Americans owe to them a great debt of gratitude, one that is only beginning to be acknowledged.

Medical Colleges for Blacks*

Howard University Medical School
  Washington, D.C. 1868
Meharry Medical School
  Nashville, TN 1876
Leonard Medical School (Shaw University)
  Raleigh, NC 1882–1914
New Orleans University Medical College, renamed Flint Medical College
  New Orleans, LA 1887–1911
Chattanooga Medical College
  Chattanooga, TN 1902
Knoxville Medical College
  Knoxville, TN 1895
University of West Tennessee College of Physicians and Surgeons
  Memphis, TN 1904–23

Total number of M.D. degrees awarded: 216

* Seven schools for blacks were established between 1868 and 1904. By 1923 only two approved schools existed, Howard and Meharry.

SOURCES

John Duffy, *The Healers: A History of American Medicine* (Urbana: University of Illinois Press, 1979): 260–88.

Mary Roth Walsh, *"Doctors Wanted: No Women Need Apply": Sexual Barriers in the Medical Profession, 1835–1925* (New Haven CT: Yale University Press, 1977), 179, 180–83.

Herbert M. Morais, *The History of the Negro in Medicine* (New York: Association for the Study of Afro-American Life and History, 1967), 57–67.

NOTES

1. Dorothy Sterling, ed., *We Are Your Sisters: Black Women in the Nineteenth Century* (New York: W. W. Norton & Company, 1984), 450.
2. Mary Roth Walsh, *"Doctors Wanted: No Women Need Apply": Sexual Barriers in the Medical Profession, 1835–1975* (New Haven, CT: Yale University Press, 1977), 194, 225, 236–37; M. O. Bousfield, "An Account of Physicians of Color in the United States," *Bulletin of the History of Medicine* 17 (January 1945): 62, 70, 80; E. Richard Brown, *Rockefeller Medicine Men: Medicine and Capitalism in America* (Berkeley: University of California Press, 1979), 88, 153; Paul Starr, *The Social Transformation of American Medicine: The Rise of a Sovereign Profession and the Making of a Vast Industry* (New York: Basic Books, 1982), 124–25.
3. Bettina Aptheker, "Quest for Dignity: Black Women in the Professions, 1885–1900," in her *Woman's Legacy: Essays on Race, Sex, and Class in American History* (Amherst: University of Massachusetts Press, 1982), 97–98; Sara W. Brown, "Colored Women Physicians," *Southern Workman* 52 (1923): 586; Sterling, *We Are Your Sisters*, 440–41; Leslie L. Alexander, "Early Medical Heroes: Susan Smith McKinney Steward, M.D., 1847–1918: First Afro-American Woman Phy-

sician in New York State," *Journal of the National Medical Association* 67 (March 1975): 173–75.

4. Walsh, *"Doctors Wanted,"* 186; Cora Bagley Marrett, "On the Evolution of Women's Medical Societies," *Bulletin of the History of Medicine* 53 (1979): 434.

5. Bousfield, "An Account of Physicians of Color," 592; Numa P. G. Adams, "Sources of Supply of Negro Health Personnel: Section A: Physicians," *Journal of Negro Education* 6 (July 1937): 468.

6. *Medical and Surgical Observer* (October 1893): 184. M. Vandahurst Lynk was the editor of this first black medical journal. He also founded the medical department of the University of West Tennessee in Memphis.

7. Rayford W. Logan, *Howard University: The First Hundred Years, 1867–1967* (New York: New York University Press, 1969), 42, 47.

8. Daniel Smith Lamb, *Howard University Medical Department: A Historical, Biographical and Statistical Souvenir* (Washington, D.C.: R. Beresford, 1900), 142; Brown, "Colored Women Physicians," 592; Bousfield, "An Account of Physicians of Color," 70; Aptheker, *Woman's Legacy,* 100; *Catalogue of Officers and Students of Howard University, 1971–1872,* 54, 62.

9. Cited in Herbert M. Morais, *The History of the Negro in Medicine* (New York: Association for the Study of Negro Life and History, 1967), 43; *Catalogue of the Officers and Students of Howard University from March 1887 to March 1879,* 12–13. All Catalogues found in the Moorland-Spingarn Library of Howard University, Washington, D.C.

10. Morais, *The History of the Negro in Medicine,* 43; Logan, *Howard University,* 47.

11. James Summerville, *Educating Black Doctors: A History of Meharry College* (University, AL: The University of Alabama Press, 1983), 31–32; Darlene Clark Hine, "The Pursuit of Professional Equality: Meharry Medical College, 1921–1938, A Case Study," *New Perspectives in Black Educational History,* Vincent P. Franklin and James D. Anderson, ed, (Boston: G. K. Hall, 1978), 173–92.

12. Charles Victor Roman, *Meharry Medical College: A History* (Nashville, TN: Sunday School Publishing Board of the National Baptist Convention, 1934), 64, 76, 107; Summerville, *Educating Black Doctors,* 33.

13. Walsh, *"Doctors Wanted",* 62, 181, 195.

14. Aptheker, *Woman's Legacy,* 98–99; Sterling, *We Are Your Sisters,* 443–49; Brown, "Colored Women Physicians," 591; Margaret Jerrido, "Black Women Physicians: A Triple Burden," *Alumnae News,* The Woman's Medical College of Pennsylvania, now the Medical College of Pennsylvania (Summer 1979): 45; Ruth Abram, "Daughters of Aesculapius," *Alumnae News,* The Woman's Medical College of Pennsylvania, now the Medical College of Pennsylvania (Fall 1983): 10.

15. E. Wilber Block, "Farmer's Daughter Effect: The Case of the Negro Female Professional," *Phylon* 30 (Spring 1969): 17–26; Elizabeth R. Haynes, "Negroes in Domestic Service in the United States," *Journal of Negro History* 8 (1923): 422–28; Lawrence B. de Graff, "Race, Sex and Region: Black Women in the American West," *Pacific Historical Review* 49 (May 1980): 285–313.

16. G. R. Richings, *Evidences of Progress Among Colored People* (Philadelphia: George S. Ferguson Co., 1905), 412; L. A. Scruggs, *Women of Distinction: Remarkable in Works and Invincible in Character* (Raleigh, NC: L. A. Scruggs, 1982), 177–78; Matthew Anderson, *Presbyterianism: Its Relation to the Negro* (Philadelphia: John McGill, White & Company, 1899), contains sketches of the Berean Church, Caroline Still Wiley Anderson, and the author; Brown, "Colored Women Physicians," 585.

17. Brown, "Colored Women Physicians," 591; Richings, *Evidences of Progress,* 411–12.

18. Richings, *Evidences of Progress,* 411–12; Brown, "Colored Women Physicians," 585–86.
19. Sterling, *We Are Your Sisters,* 441–43; Scruggs, *Women of Distinction,* 100–103.
20. Brown, "Colored Women Physicians," 588; Aptheker, *Woman's Legacy,* 98; Elizabeth L. Davis, *Lifting As They Climb: The National Association of Colored Women* (Washington, D.C.: National Association of Colored Women's Clubs, 1933), 292; Sterling, *We Are Your Sisters,* 443–448.
21. Quoted in Sterling's *We Are Your Sisters,* 445–46; Richings, *Evidences of Progress,* 413; Scruggs, *Women of Distinction,* 364–65; Brown, "Colored Women Physicians," 591.
22. Quoted in Charlayne Hunter-Gault's "Black Women M.D.'s: Spirit and Endurance," *The New York Times,* November 16, 1977.
23. Ibid.
24. Bousfield, "An Account of Physicians of Color," 72; E. H. Beardsley, "Making Separate Equal: Black Physicians and the Problems of Medical Segregation in the Pre-World War II South," *Bulletin of the History of Medicine* 57 (Fall 1983): 382–96.
25. Sterling, *We Are Your Sisters,* 444–45.
26. Elizabeth Blackwell, *Pioneer Work in Opening the Medical Profession to Women: Autobiographical Sketches* (New York: Schocken Books, 1977 reprint of 1895 edition), 228; Jerrido, "Black Women Physicians," 4–5.
27. *Directory of the Philanthropic, Educational and Religious Association of Churches of Philadelphia,* 2nd ed. (Lancaster, PA: New Era Printing Company, 1903), 158; Philadelphia City Hall, Wills. Inventory and Appraisement, filed, January 11, 1923; Sterling, *We Are Your Sisters,* 440–41; Brown, "Colored Women Physicians," 586.
28. Anderson, *Presbyterianism: Its Relation to the Negro,* 5ff; Margaret Jerrido, "In Recognition of Early Black Women Physicians," *Women and Health* 5 (Fall 1980): 1–3.
29. Aptheker, *Woman's Legacy,* 98, 99, 101; *Atlanta University Bulletin,* November 1891.
30. Logan, *Howard University,* 136; Brown, "Colored Women Physicians," 589–90; Aptheker, *Woman's Legacy,* 99.
31. Scruggs, *Women of Distinction,* 267–68.
32. Sister M. Anthony Scally, *Medicine, Motherhood and Mercy: the Story of a Black Woman Doctor* (Washington, D.C.: Associated Publisher, 1979), 23–27.
33. Isabella Vandervall, "Some Problems of the Colored Woman Physician," *The Woman's Medical Journal* 27 (July 1917): 156–58.
34. Aptheker, *Woman's Legacy,* 99.
35. Quoted in Sterling's *We Are Your Sisters,* 440, 441, 443.
36. Scruggs, *Women of Distinction,* 100–103, 177–78; Brown, "Colored Women Physicians," 585.
37. Maritcha Lyons, "Dr. Susan S. McKinney Steward," *Homespun Heroines and Other Women of Distinction,* Hallie Quinn Brown, editor (Xenia, Ohio, Aldine Publishing Company, 1926; reprint 1971), 162; Alexander, "Early Medical Heroes: Susan Smith McKinney Steward," 21–23; Davis, *Lifting As They Climb,* 292; Sterling, *We Are Your Sisters, 440–43;* William Peper, "Boro Had 1st Negro Woman M.D. in 1870s," the *Sun,* May 9, 1960; Brooklyn *Times,* June 27, 1891.
38. Scruggs, *Women of Distinction,* 267–68.
39. Brooklyn *Times,* June 27, 1891; Scruggs, *Women of Distinction,* 267–68.
40. Brown, "Colored Women Physicians," 582.

Every Woman is a Nurse

Work and Gender in the Emergence of Nursing

BARBARA MELOSH

WOMEN'S dominance in nursing is nearly as strong as our monopoly on motherhood: nursing has always been a woman's job. In the mid-nineteenth century, most nursing care was done at home as part of women's domestic duties. Florence Nightingale's 1860 manual, *Notes on Nursing,* was addressed to women in families and opened with the assertion, "Every woman is a nurse."[1] As medical care became more complex and more tied to hospitals, nursing gradually separated from the sphere of women's domestic work and became established as paid work that required special training. Arguments of women's special fitness for nursing connected traditional domestic roles to female participation in this new category of paid labor. As one doctor wrote in 1925, "A hospital is a home for the sick, and there can be no home unless there is a woman at the head of it."[2] While these sentimental images of nursing service lingered, the actual content and practice of nursing grew increasingly specialized. In the esoteric technological setting of modern hospitals, no one would proclaim that every woman is a nurse. But the cultural ideology of woman's place still informs the division of labor in health care: nearly every nurse is a woman.

Unlike most women's jobs, nursing has been characterized by the presence of an articulate and self-conscious elite. Beginning in 1873, they opened hospitals, arguing that nursing was a special skill that required such training.

121

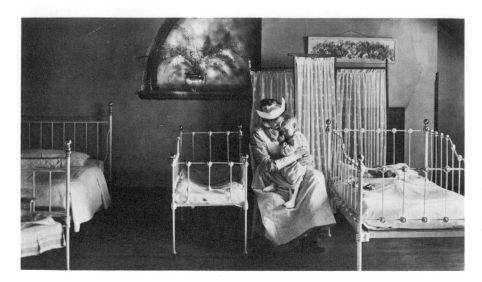

Nurse and child in Children's Ward, Northwestern Hospital (c. 1900). Minnesota Historical Society.

They struggled to establish nursing as respectable work for middle-class women, recruiting among them to replace the socially marginal women who had traditionally done most of the hospital's work. They formed associations to share their problems and to promote the cause of the "trained nurse" to a wider audience. They sought state licensure to affirm and defend the nurse's skills. In their efforts to establish educational credentials, licensure, and employment standards, they worked to assert the control over training and practice that is the mark of established professions.

Nursing leaders faced formidable obstacles in their quest for the privileges of professional status. First, the economics of health care powerfully shaped the structure of nursing. Nursing schools expanded rapidly between 1890 and 1920 because hospital administrators benefited from the unpaid labor of apprentice student nurses. Private duty nursing, the predominant form of practice before 1940, suffered the uncertain fortunes of the market: fee-for-service practice, the touted source of physicians' autonomy, often meant sparse employment, poor working conditions, exhaustion, isolation, and menial duties for nurses who cared for one patient at home or in the hospital. In its early year, public health nursing gave nurses a rare autonomy on the job; but by 1940 changing patterns of funding favored hospital-based care, and nurses lost their control of this separate domain of community health. In hospitals, nurses benefited from a growing demand for nursing services after 1940, and most became regular staff nurses with the advantages of institutional employment—more secure work, camaraderie on the job, a place in a prestigious realm of expanding medical science and technology—along with its disadvantages—low pay, a quickened work pace, little authority combined with much responsibility. Second, nursing leaders sought professionalization against considerable division in their own ranks. Many nurses resisted leaders' efforts to regulate education and practice through the strategies of increasing educational requirements and licensure.

Finally, as women workers in a "woman's" job, nurses sought control over their work against the constraints of sexism. On one hand, they drew on the strengths of separatism: their schools and, before 1940, often their hospitals, were female worlds. On the other, they experienced the disabilities of sex segregation. As leaders worked to establish nurses' training in the last quarter of the nineteenth century, they had to struggle against the idea that any woman could nurse, simply by virtue of her womanhood, arguing instead that their work required special skills and training. Even after 1940, in a situation of severe labor shortage, nurses were underpaid compared to men with equivalent education and experience. Despite nurses' skills and increasingly sophisticated training, the association of nursing with women meant that the work itself was often undervalued by physicians, patients, and the lay public.

The early years of nursing vividly illustrate these themes. Nurses' training began as a project of reform-minded women who worked to improve hospital care as part of the traditional benevolent mission of upper-class women. Inspired by Florence Nightingale's work in England, women in the United States organized the first three training schools in 1873, at Bellevue Hospital in New York, Massachusetts General Hospital in Boston, and Connecticut Hospital in New Haven. The idea of a training course for nurses spread slowly, and "trained nurses," graduates of these early hospital courses, were a rarity. In 1880, the U.S. Census listed 13,000 women who nursed for hire; only an estimated 560 of those were graduates of hospital courses. In 1890, thirty-five schools were operating.[3]

Between 1890 and 1920, broad changes in medical care created new opportunities for the trained nurse and supported the emergence of nursing as a respectable occupation for women. New medical knowledge placed nursing skills on a more scientific basis; for example, as antisepsis and asepsis became widely accepted by the end of the nineteenth century, doctors saw the advantages of a better educated hospital attendant. Other social changes also influenced the laywoman's displacement by a paid nurse. Historian Morris Vogel has suggested that newly isolated middle-class families began to hire private duty nurses for home care and to resort more often to hospital care as urban life disrupted the old resources of extended families.[4] Meanwhile, as historian David Rosner demonstrates, urban growth spurred hospital expansion and reorganization.[5] As the pace of industrial work quickened and an influx of new immigrants arrived in American cities, workplace injuries increased and a larger working-class population strained the limited resources of nineteenth-century hospitals. Finally, in the late nineteenth century, medical practice began to shift from the home to the hospital. With more reliable antisepsis and asepsis, the terrible postsurgical mortality rates of the nineteenth century fell, and surgical intervention increased dramatically. Offering new opportunities to medical practitioners, hospitals became laboratories for experimental techniques, treatments, and research.

Once scarce and widely scattered, hospitals became a commonplace feature of urban and suburban landscapes. In 1873, when the first nursing school was founded, there were fewer than 200 hospitals in the United States. By 1910, over 4,000 were open, and less than two decades later, 7,416 were offering their services.[6] From the charitable institutions of Nightingale's day, hospitals were becoming centers for a prestigious and profitable service industry.

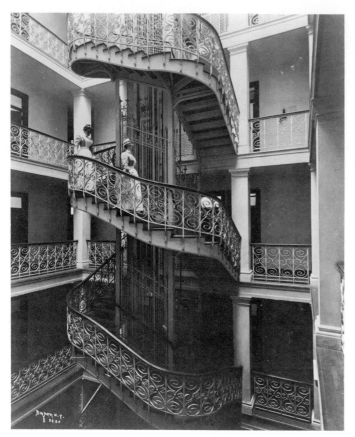

Nurses descending stairs, St. Luke's Hospital (1899). Museum of the City of New York.

Hospital expansion provided the economic motivation and bases for the establishment of hundreds of new training schools for nurses. Nursing schools opened all over the country as hospital administrators sought a more disciplined work force and wooed a fee-paying clientele by replacing attendants with respectable student nurses. By 1910, one in four hospitals had nursing schools, and in 1927, 2,155 hospitals kept their wards supplied with student nurses.[7]

This burgeoning growth was a decidedly mixed blessing. On one hand, hospital development assured the expansion of nursing schools and promoted the acceptance of the "trained nurse" as superior to the many attendants for hire who cared for the sick without the benefit of any formal course of education; on the other, the economic structure of hospital schools imposed limitations on nurses' education and quickly created an employment crisis of major proportions. Before 1940, hospitals did not routinely hire graduate nurses, the products of their own schools, to work on the wards. Instead, hospitals replenished their work forces by recruiting new crops of students, who handled the ward work under the supervision of only a few graduate nurses. The result was that, between 1900 and 1920, the number of trained nurses rose from 11,804 to 149,128, while the population of the United States increased by less than 50 percent.[8] Even in the context of rapidly increasing demand for medical and nursing services, this flood of new nurses could not be absorbed. A few graduates found supervisory jobs in hospitals, and still fewer moved into the small new field of public health. But most graduated from their schools to work in the uncertain freelance market of private-duty nursing. Before World War I, there were already ominous signs of the collapse of the private duty market, and by 1920 many nurses were struggling desperately for work. Meanwhile, the expanding hospitals cried out for more nurses—and continued to recruit students to fill the need.

Deeply concerned about the uncontrolled expansion of nursing, leaders tried to raise the standards of admission and reorganize the training courses so that the ward work occupied less of the students' time. But their efforts met strong resistance. Most physicians believed that current training was adequate, and some felt threatened by the prospect of better-educated nurses. Hospital administrators, many of them nurses themselves, had strong economic and ideological commitments to the apprenticeship system: they benefited from the labor of student nurses and often believed that on-the-job training was the most important part of the nurses' education, fearing that higher standards or a system of state licensure might devalue their own training or put them out of work altogether.

In the end, the crisis in nursing was resolved largely by forces beyond nurses' control or direction. The shortage of hospital, medical, and nursing services during World War II heightened public concern about health care. In the postwar years, new federal funding and expanded private insurance plans underwrote hospital construction, educational subsidies, and patient care. Meanwhile, the growing specialization of medicine, the increasing use of hospital based technologies, and the rising cost of nursing services all contributed to the decline of private duty care. Nursing's market crisis was reversed by the tremendous expansion of hospital facilities after World War II and by new patterns of hiring that brought graduate nurses into hospital staff positions. Although, as Linda Aiken has shown, nurses' salaries remained depressed even in the situation of chronic labor shortage that prevailed from World War II until very recently,[9] nonetheless the demand for nurses brought generous educational subsidies, some improvements in working conditions, and perhaps a larger measure of public recognition for the skill of nursing.

At first glance, the histories of nurses and female doctors would appear to have little in common. While nurses faced the problems of women workers in a female occupation, women doctors sought entrance to a determinedly male profession. Even as nursing found its place in the hospital division of labor, female doctors were increasingly constrained by the tightening boundaries of medical professionalization.

From these different positions, though, both women in nursing and women in medicine experienced the hazards of professionalization in a society of unequal gender relations. For nurses, the power and autonomy of full professionalization would remain elusive: that position is reserved for the most privileged of occupations, and in a sexist and racist society, such jobs are mostly reserved for white males. The history of female doctors illustrates the contradictory results of separatism: they would win a modicum of success partly because late-nineteenth-century ideology defined women and children

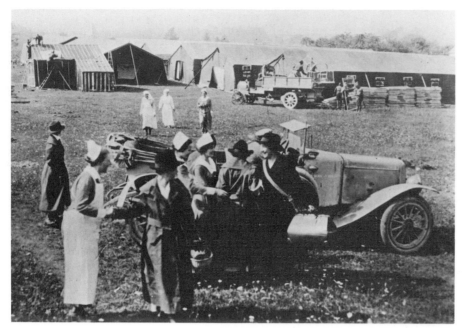

Nurses from the New York Infirmary in France during World War I. New York Infirmary/Beekman Downtown Hospital.

as a special class of patients better served by female physicians. But as the ideology of professionalization—including an ideology of objectivity that denied the argument of women's special fitness or needs—took firmer hold in medicine, women doctors lost their precarious hold.[10]

The contemporary situation illustrates both change and persistence in the institutions and ideology of American gender relationships. Although many observers point to the large number of female medical students—one third or more of some entering classes—as evidence of the success of the twentieth-century women's movement, it is worth observing that the barriers against women have eased at a time when the medical profession is entering a period of relative decline. Some have noted an oversupply of physicians—that is, too many doctors to sustain the high incomes and diverse opportunities that have made the profession so attractive. At the same time, the celebrated autonomy of the profession has eroded somewhat under consumer revolts, pressure for cost containment, and growing state regulation. In what measure is women's increasing representation in medicine a feminist victory? To what extent might it reflect male flight from a declining profession?

Nursing, by contrast, has remained remarkably stable as a female occupation: male nurses have never represented more than 5 percent of the total. Nursing is a good job for a woman—it offers more satisfaction and better pay than many women's jobs. But the absence of men in nursing attests to its disadvantaged position in the whole labor market: nurses' incomes and authority are simply not commensurate with their education, skills, and responsibilities. Ironically, as nursing leaders have struggled for professionalization they may have inadvertently exacerbated this imbalance: these reformers have been more successful in raising educational requirements than in im-

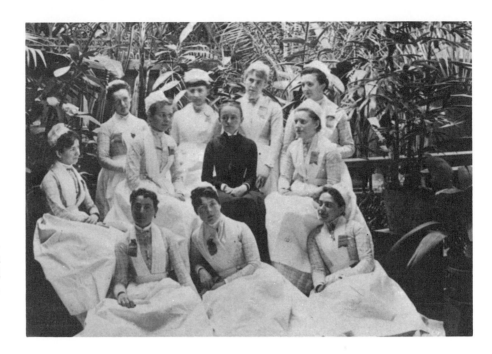

Student nurses (c. 1890). Medical Archives, New York Hospital, Cornell Medical Center.

proving wages and working conditions. In the current situation of cost containment, declining hospital use, and uncertainty about nurses' place in the future organization of health care, it will not be easy to overcome this legacy of sexual inequality.

The comparison between women in nursing and medicine suggests both the gains of the women's movement and the road we have yet to travel. Exceptional women now do appear to enjoy an expanded field of opportunity; some have found their way into privileged positions as liberal feminism makes inroads. But it will take a broader commitment to equality to establish principles of comparable worth. As many nurses recognize, nursing's future is inextricably linked with the future of the women's movement.

NOTES

1. Florence Nightingale, *Notes on Nursing: What It Is, and What It Is Not* (New York: Appleton, 1860), 3.
2. Alfred Worcester, *Nurses and Nursing* (Cambridge, MA: Harvard University Press, 1927), 9.
3. May Ayres Burgess, *Nurses, Patients, and Pocketbooks: Report of a Study of the Economics of Nursing* (New York: Committee on the Grading of Nursing Schools, 1928), 40.
4. Morris J. Vogel, *The Invention of the Modern Hospital, Boston, 1870–1930* (Chicago: University of Chicago Press, 1980), 99–101.
5. David Rosner, *A Once Charitable Enterprise: Hospitals and Health Care in Brooklyn and New York, 1885–1915* (Cambridge, MA: Cambridge University Press, 1982); see esp. ch. 1, "Health Care and Community Change," 13–35.
6. E. H. L. Corwin, *The American Hsopital* (New York: The Commonwealth Fund,

1946), 6–8; Paul Starr, "Medicine, Economy and Society in Nineteenth-Century America," *Journal of Social History* 10 (Summer 1977): 588–607; see esp. p. 598; and Starr, *The Social Transformation of American Medicine: The Rise of a Sovereign Profession and the Making of a Vast Industry*, (New York: Basic Books, 1982), 169–79.

7. Burgess, *Nurses, Patients,* 35.

8. Ibid., 35–37.

9. Linda Aiken, "The Impact of Federal Health Policy on Nurses," in idem, ed., *Nursing in the 1980s: Crises, Opportunities, Challenges* (Philadelphia: J. B. Lippincott, 1982), 3–20.

10. For two different interpretations of the history of women in medicine, see Mary Roth Walsh, *"Doctors Wanted: No Women Need Apply": Sexual Barriers in the Medical Profession, 1835–1975* (New Haven, CT: Yale University Press, 1977), and Virginia Drachman, *Hospital with a Heart: Women Doctors and the Paradox of Separatism at the New England Hospital, 1862–1969* (Ithaca, NY: Cornell University Press, 1984).

Part Three

HER CALLING IN LIFE

The Class of 1879 of the Woman's Medical College of Pennsylvania

The . . . physician is not debating in her own mind whether she shall next turn her attention to the study of music or of literature, or it may be of telegraphy. She has found her calling in life; it is soul-satisfying.
—Dr. Rachel Bodley, Dean
Woman's Medical College of Pennsylvania 1881

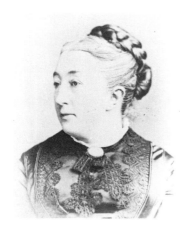

Dr. Rachel Bodley, 1831–1888,
ASCWM, MCP.

Introduction

THE nineteenth-century women's medical movement was blessed with leaders of heroic proportion. But it was their followers, the "ordinary" women physicians, whose collective character, training, failures, and successes would determine the fate of the nascent movement for women in medicine. It is to this "typical" woman physician that our attention now turns. Who was she? How was she trained?

The twenty members of the Class of 1879 of the Woman's Medical College of Pennsylvania, most of whom commenced their medical training in the nation's centennial year, serve as prototypes for all late-nineteenth-century women doctors.

They graduated on Thursday, March 13, 1879. The Philadelphia *Evening Bulletin* reported that promptly at noon, Association Hall in Philadelphia was "completely filled with gentlemen and lady friends of the students and graduates" of the Woman's Medical College of Pennsylvania, describing further,

> The sides and corners of the platform were adorned with wide spreading palms and the front encircled with a profusion of floral offerings. . . . After the performance of choice musical selections by Carl Sentz's Orchestra . . . the exercises were opened by the entrance of the corporators and faculty of the college . . . followed by the graduates, who proceeded to the places reserved for them in front of the audience.

After a brief prayer by the Reverend Dr. Kellog and an orchestral rendition of Verdi's "The Angel's Prayer," Mr. Morris Perot, Esq., took up his "pleasing duty, as President of the Board, of conferring the degrees." The names of the twenty graduates were posted in the Philadelphia papers, grouped by home state:

131

Pennsylvania: Sarah A. Cohen, Phoebe H. Flagler, Agnes Kemp, Anna S. Kugler, Ida E. Richardson, Almina F. Rhodes, Louise Schneider
New Jersey: Harriet G. Belcher, H. Louisa Exton
New York: Martha M. Dunn, Eleanor E. Galt, Sophia E. Howard, Mina Fitch Wood
New Hampshire: Mary Alice Avery
Rhode Island: Lucy R. Weaver
Vermont: Julia P. Pease
Illinois: Emma A. Baldwin, Rachel J. Nicol
Ohio: Sophia Presley
Massachusetts: Mary H. Wolfenden

The Philadelphia *Evening Bulletin* went on to declare that of all the people to receive the M.D. degree that week, for this was commencement week in Philadelphia, "none [was] so interesting as the little band of a score of women who [went] out from the Woman's Medical College to take their places in the profession of medicine."

The "interesting little band" was typical of the type of women who, in the late nineteenth century, sought medical careers. Hailing primarily from large families living in small towns in the northeastern states, they were the daughters of farmers and artisans (not infrequently immigrants). Generally educated in private schools or female seminaries, many had worked as teachers or homemakers prior to entering medical school at an average age of thirty.

Here, in the statistics of which their dean, Dr. Rachel Bodley, would have approved, are the particulars of the members of the class:

Birthplace of Parents
United States 11
Europe 7
Unknown 2

Occupation of Fathers
Artisan/tradesman 7
Farmer 4
Business 3
Minister 2
Professional 2
Unknown 2

Education Prior to Medical School
Normal schools/female seminaries 9
Public school 3
College 2
Unknown 6

Occupation Prior to Medical School
Teacher 6
Domestic 5
Unknown 8

Age Upon Entering Medical School
19–25 7
26–30 4
31–40 6
Over 40 3

Marriage and Children
Married 11 (of the 11, 2 divorced)
Married with children 9
Never married 9
Unknown 1

Occupation of Husbands
Professional 4 (3 physicians)
Business 2
Farmer 2
Minister 1
Unknown 2

Age at Death
Under 50 4
50–60 3
61–70 4
71–80 5
Over 80 3
Unknown 1

Yearbook: The Class of '79

Dr. Mary Alice Avery, 1849–1904.

The second of seven children in a farming family, Mary Alice taught school for eight years after graduating from the New Hampton Literary Institution (New Hampton, New Hampshire). In 1885, the superintendent of the Philadelphia Hospital commended her for bravery after she rescued a patient in the Insane Department during a fire. Upon her death, her colleagues eulogized her: "To how many homes has she brought solace and courage, to how many hearts new life and hope."

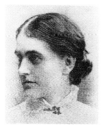

Bowdoin College Library.

Dr. Emma A. Baldwin, 1840–1905.

Emma entered the Woman's Medical College of Pennsylvania after studying at the Chicago Hospital for Women and Children. Returning to Chicago after graduation, she obtained housing near the hospital and worked as a dispensary physician. Her career after 1890 remains a mystery. She died in Eureka Springs, Arkansas.

Dr. Harriet G. Belcher, 1842–1887.

The eldest of four children born to a New Jersey factory owner, Harriet cared for her siblings after her mother's death in 1863. She entered medical school

133

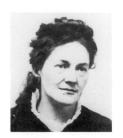

Dr. Harriet G. Belcher, 1842–87 (c. 1880). Santa Barbara Historical Society; gift of Mrs. Alan McCone.

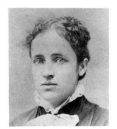

ASCWM, MCP.; gift of Morris B. Abram.

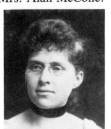

Corey Family Collection.

in 1875 over her father's objections. Deciding that her "rather heterodox religious opinions" disqualified her from a career as a medical missionary, she opened a private practice in Providence, Rhode Island. Three years later, she moved to the new resort town of Santa Barbara, California and could soon report, "My success is assured."

Dr. Sarah A. Cohen (May), 1857–1934.

The third of four children born to immigrant Jewish parents, Sarah attended medical school after her father's death and over her mother's violent objections. Upon graduation, she practiced in Philadelphia with her elder brother, a graduate of Jefferson Medical College, and her younger brother, a pharmacist. Neither her marriage to a shoe store owner in 1892 nor the births of her two children interrupted her medical career. In 1903, she graduated in the third class of the Philadelphia College of Osteopathy and thereafter combined regular therapeutics with osteopathic techniques.

Dr. Martha M. Dunn (Corey), 1852–1927.

Orphaned at an early age, Martha grew up in the home of a Baptist minister and his wife in Evans, New York. After attending private academies in upstate New York, Martha entered the homeopathic Women's Medical College of New York. In 1877, listing Dr. Cornelia Green, founder of the famed Castile Sanitorium, as her preceptor, Martha switched to the Woman's Medical College of Pennsylvania. In 1887, she sailed to England to study with the noted surgeon and antivivesectionist Dr. Lawson Tait. Marriage in 1888 was followed by the birth of three sons. Deserted by her husband shortly after the birth of their third child, Martha moved her family to La Jolla, California, and established a thriving practice.

Dr. Henrietta L. Exton, 1843–1907

Born in Union, New Jersey, to a family whose American roots reached back to the Revolution, Henrietta grew up on the family's prosperous Hunterdon County farm. Although she applied for a medical license in 1885, there is no evidence that she practiced medicine after graduation. However, she was quite active in the antivivisection movement and in the Society for the Prevention of Cruelty to Animals. (Her will made specific provisions for her pet sheep.) The farm handyman remembered Henrietta, a member of the Colonial Dames, as "quiet, refined, and unobtrusive. It was her daily chore to make my bed."

Dr. Phoebe H. Flager (Hagenbuch), 1832–1927

Raised in a Quaker home in Stroudsburg, Pennsylvania, Phoebe was twice married by the time she entered medical school. Her second husband, a drover of a "somewhat peculiar bent," died during Phoebe's medical studies. After working as a private practitioner in Bryan, Ohio, and Williamsport, Pennsylvania—along the way marrying and divorcing a druggist—Phoebe returned to her hometown and developed a loyal following. Her grandson remembers that her homemade remedy for poison ivy was particularly effective. She routinely gathered her own herbs for her medicines.

Dr. Eleanor E. Galt (Simmons), 1854–1909.

The daughter of a Delaware County, New York, physician, Eleanor was privately educated. Upon graduation from medical school, she worked at the Nursery and Child's Hospital in Staten Island, New York, and later opened a private practice in Elizabeth, New Jersey. Her marriage in 1890 to an attorney resulted in a move to Coconut Grove, Florida, where she conducted a private practice and participated actively in community affairs. The House-keepers' Club, of which she was a member, benefited often from her lectures and from her recipe for green mango pie.

Dr. Sophia E. Howard, 1844–1893.

The *Fairport Herald Mail* reported on Sophia's graduation from medical school with delight, saying that her many friends would be "pleased to hear of her having acquired a thorough knowledge of the profession." The daughter of a carriage maker, Sophia was educated at the progressive Howland School in Union Springs, New York. Rachel Bodley, who would serve as dean of the Woman's Medical College of Pennsylvania, was at the time a lecturer on chemistry and botany at the school. A temperance advocate, Sophia lectured before junior members of the Women's Christian Temperance Union while carrying on a private practice in Auburn, New York.

Dr. Agnes Nininger Kemp, 1823–1908.

One of nine children born to a Harrisburg, Pennsylvania, victualler and his wife, Agnes was widowed as a young woman. Her second marriage resulted in the births of three children, only one of whom survived to adulthood. A devout Quaker, Agnes was deeply involved in movements for kindergartens, police matrons, temperance, social purity, and suffrage. At the age of fifty-eight, she graduated from medical school. Continuing her community work, she opened a private practice and was quickly invited into the local medical society. Heartbroken over the death of her daughter, a professor at Swarthmore, Agnes died a year later.

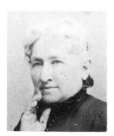

Dorothy Lawrence Collection.

135

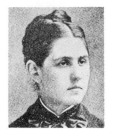

Dr. Anna S. Kugler, 1856–1930.

The second of six children born to a devout Lutheran family, Anna early determined on a career as a medical missionary. In 1882, after working under another Woman's Medical College graduate at the State Hospital for the Insane in Norristown, Pennsylvania, Anna sailed for Guntur, India, to begin her life's work. Kugler insisted that it was important that the doctor attach "as much importance to the religious teaching as to any part of the day's routine."

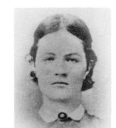

Dr. Rachel J. Nicol, 1845–1881.

The only daughter of the five children born to an Illinois farming couple, "Jennie," as she was known, was encouraged to study medicine by the husband of her best friend. A degree from Monmouth College (Jacksonville, Illinois) enabled her to complete her medical studies at an accelerated rate. Determined to deepen her knowledge, Jennie sailed to Switzerland and enrolled in the Univeristy of Zurich. There she died an untimely death from meningitis. Pi Beta Phi, the sorority she helped found, built a health clinic in her name that still operates today.

Dr. Julia P. Pease (Abbott), 1849–1919.

In her early twenties, Julia, the third of four children born to Rutland, Vermont's Congregational minister and his wife, worked as a "companion" in a neighbor's home. Soon after graduating from medical school, Julia married another physician and moved to Lawrence, Massachusetts. When the deaths of two children and the births of two others interrupted her medical practice, she worked as first vice president of the Ladies' Charitable Society to found the Lawrence General Hospital, serving on its board of trustees for twenty years.

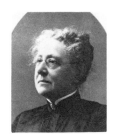

Dr. Sophia Presley, 1834–1919.

Born in Ireland, Sophia immigrated with her family to Steubenville, Ohio, where her father worked as a glass packer. Her degree from the Granville Female Seminary (Granville, Ohio) enabled her to graduate from medical school in only two years. A woman of wide community interests, she carried on a private practice in Camden while working at the City Dispensary, teaching at the New Jersey Training School for Nurses, and serving as a trustee of the West Jersey Orphanage for Colored Children. Her repeated attempts to join the local medical society met with success in 1890.

Dr. Ida E. Richardson, 1845–1902.

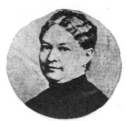

Convinced that she had received a "heaven born call," Ida enrolled in medical school after working in her father's umbrella store and as a governess with "some of the best families" of Philadelphia. Upon graduating from medical school, she opened what soon became a large private practice from her home on South 16th Street. An instructor at the Woman's Medical College of Pennsylvania, Ida helped found the West Philadelphia Hospital for Women, joined numerous medical societies, and died surrounded by her colleagues at the Woman's Hospital.

ASCWM, MCP.

Dr. Almina F. Rhodes (Dean), 1850–1897.

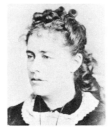

The second of six children born to a lumberman/farmer and his wife in Cambridge Springs, Pennsylvania, Almina taught in the local schools after graduating from the Normal School in Edinboro, Pennsylvania. Her interest in pedagogy found expression in her medical school thesis, "The Physician's Duty as an Educator." Upon graduation, Almina returned to her hometown and established a sanitarium, which specialized in the popular "vacuum treatment." In 1884 she married a former patient, farmer Milton Dean, by whom she had one child.

Kreitz Family Collection.

Dr. Louise Schneider (Blum), 1854–1923.

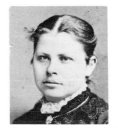

One of seven children born to German immigrants, Louise attended normal school in Philadelphia. A year's study in Zurich, Switzerland, completed her medical education. Returning to Philadelphia, Louise opened a practice from her home on Diamond Street and volunteered in a free clinic. Neither her 1882 marriage to a Moravian minister nor the 1887 birth of her only child curtailed Louise's medical career. When her husband accepted the position of headmaster of the Nazareth Military Academy, Louise served as "lady principal."

Petrulias Family Collection.

Dr. Lucy R. Weaver (Soule), 1852–1922

"Not five feet tall, her hands could not reach an octave on the piano," Lucy was the youngest of four children born in Providence, Rhode Island, to a furniture manufacturer and his wife. After graduation, Lucy returned to Providence, accompanied by her roommate, Dr. Harriet Belcher, and aided by her preceptor, surgeon Anita Tyng, M.D. In 1886, Lucy married Dr. Nicholas Emery Soule, seventeen years her senior. Two miscarriages and the birth of the couple's only child put an end to Lucy's medical career.

Dr. Mary H. Wolfenden (Battershall), 1854–1928

Born to English immigrants in New York City, Mary moved to Attleboro, Massachusetts, where her father worked in coloring. After working as a teacher, Mary studied with sanitarium founder Dr. Laura Mackie before entering medical school. After stints at the New England Hospital and the Nursery and Child's Hospital, Mary returned to Attleboro, married another physician, joined him in practice and bore a son. A member of her local medical society, Mary served as vice chairman of the Republican City Committee and worked for suffrage with the Woman's Republican Club.

Dr. Mina Fitch Wood, dates unknown.

The *Courtland Standard* in Courtland, New York, was fond of reporting on Dr. Mina B. Wood, who practiced in an office in the Courtland Standard building. Seemingly certain of community interest, the paper informed readers of the physicians's illnesses and recoveries. In the summer of 1883, the paper announced Dr. Wood was leaving to take over the supervision of a Staten Island Hospital. It carried the doctor's card, announcing the date of her intended return. In 1887, the community learned that Dr. Wood was studying microscopy in New York. Nothing is known of Mina's family or of her life after 1887.

Give Her Knowledge

The Class of 1879 in Training   RUTH J. ABRAM

Give her knowledge
commensurate with her natural qualifications;
enable her to go forth,
healing the sick and comforting the afflicted
and she will bless the world
—Annual Announcement, Woman's Medical College of Pennsylvania, 1851

IN 1850, the Woman's Medical College of Pennsylvania opened its doors in the back of a rented house on Arch Street in Philadelphia. So came into being the first medical college for women in the world. From the beginning, it promised to confer a medical degree that would "not be inferior to those of the graduates of any other medical institution of this country or in Europe."[1] Throughout the nineteenth century, aware that the entire concept of the medical education of women was on trial and anxious to distinguish itself, the college did offer a superior course, often initiating groundbreaking reforms. Operating under intense public scrutiny, professors (male and female) were careful to teach only regular therapeutics. They stressed practical training long before it was common to do so. To this end, a college-affiliated dispensary and hospital were opened in 1858 and 1861 respectively, and in 1869 the "Progressive Course" was introduced. This

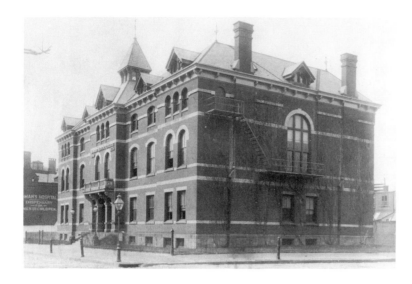

The Woman's Medical College of Pennsylvania, North College Avenue, 1875–1929 (1880s. ASCWM, MCP.

revised curriculum featured a longer course of study, freeing students for more comprehensive practical training and offering alternatives to the preceptor system, in which a student's education was limited by the proficiency of the private practitioner with whom she studied (if she could find one at all). Harvard Medical School's adoption of the Progressive Course in 1873 underscored its success.

In addition to the skills they acquired at the lectures, clinics, and demonstrations, nineteenth-century students at the Woman's Medical College learned a humanistic attitude. In 1874, Dr. Sarah A. Dolley told her pupils to regard the patient as "something more than a static entity . . . whose muscles, nerves, and joints are not simply a bundle of levers, pulleys, and hinges but . . . the instruments of that mysterious something we call life."[2]

Life—intellectual, professional, social—was full for the students at the Woman's Medical College in the late nineteenth century, as the memorabilia that follow amply illustrate. Animated by the prospect of worthy and rewarding service as women doctors in what has been referred to as the "golden era" of women in medicine, members of the Class of '79 undertook their studies with great expectations of the day when they too could "go forth" and "bless the world" with their healing powers.

Building

In 1875 the Woman's Medical College dedicated a new building on North College Avenue, the first building ever constructed expressly for the medical education of women. The college was located at this site from 1876 to 1929, when it moved to its present site on Henry Avenue.

This new building is a fine one, very completely arranged; and fitted up.
–Harriet Belcher, 1876.

Faculty

I am highly pleased with the Medical College so far. . . . Some of the professors make themselves quite intelligible and others have given five or six lectures without using a single word by means of which we could gain the slightest clue to enable us to guess what they were talking about. . . . The professor in physiology, after the quiz yesterday, complimented the class on the amount of information we [had] acquired.
—Rachel Nicol, 1876

The corps of professors is very pleasant . . . some of them lecturing on the same points for Jefferson College or the University.
—Harriet Belcher, 1875

Students

There is quite a large class of students, most of them refined, earnest, cultivated women. There are some strange looking specimens, but very few.
—Harriet Belcher, 1875

Academic Standards

The Woman's Medical College upheld standards as rigorous as those of the most prominent regular medical schools.

Requirements for Graduation. Twenty-seventh Annual Announcement, Woman's Medical College of Pennsylvania, 1876–77. ASCWM, MCP.

REQUIREMENTS FOR GRADUATION.

1. The candidate must have obtained the age of twenty one years, and must possess creditable literary attainments.

2. The candidate must have been engaged in the study of medicine for three years; and, during at least two years of that time, either the private pupil of a respectable practitioner of medicine or the Special Student of the College.*

Six months of medical service in a recognized hospital will be considered equivalent to one year's private or college preceptorship; not, however, to abate from the three years of required medical study.

3. The candidate must have attended two courses of Lectures on the following subjects:

Chemistry and Toxicology.
Anatomy.
Materia Medica and General Therapeutics.
Physiology and Hygiene.
Principles and Practice of Medicine.
Principles and Practice of Surgery,
Obstetrics and Diseases of Women and Children.

The two courses of lectures must have been attended in different years, and one at least in this College. The candidate must also have taken instruction in Practical Anatomy, equivalent in amount to one disection of all the usual divisions of the subject.

4. The application for the Degree must be made six weeks before the close of the session. The candidate, at the time of application, must exhibit to the Dean evidence of having complied with the above requirements; she must also present the graduation fee, and a thesis of her own composition and penmanship, on some subject which has direct application to medicine.

To such students as attend three sessions or more, the option is offered of the division of the final examination for the Degree of Doctor of Medicine as follows:

* See College preceptorship, p. 11.

Terms. Twenty-seventh Annual Announcement, Woman's Medical College of Pennsylvania, 1876–77. ASCWM, MCP.

Classwork

At an average age of thirty and seasoned by life experience, members of the Woman's Medical College Class of 1879 approached this opportunity to develop the skills to earn a livelihood with seriousness of purpose not infrequently joined by a well-honed sense of humor.

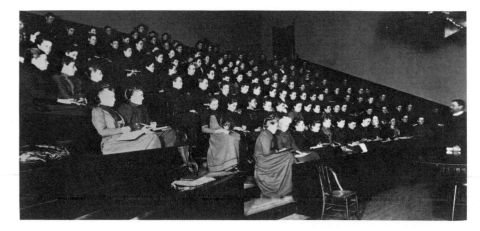

Lecture hall, Woman's Medical College of Pennsylvania (c. 1890). ASCWM, MCP.

Woman's Medical College of Pennsylvania.

North College Avenue and 21st Street, Philadelphia.

WINTER SESSION—1876-77.

ORDER OF LECTURES AND CLINICS.

Hours.	Monday.	Tuesday.	Wednesday.	Thursday.	Friday.	Saturday.
10 A. M.	Chemistry.	Pennsylvania Hospital Clinics.	Chemistry.	Practice.	Chemistry.	Practice.
11 "	Obstetrics.		Obstetrics.	Materia Medica.	Obstetrics.	Materia Medica.
12 "	Woman's Hospital Medical Clinic.		Materia Medica.	Woman's Hospital Surgical Clinic.	Surgery.	Woman's Hospital Obstetrical Clinic.
3 P. M.	Physiology.	Surgery.	Physiology.	Surgery.	Physiology.	
4 "	Anatomy.	Practice.	Anatomy.		Anatomy.	
7½ "				Histology.		

EXAMINATIONS UPON LECTURES.

9 A. M.			Chemistry.			Materia Medica.
5 P. M.	Anatomy.	Practice.	Surgery.	Obstetrics.	Physiology.	

WOMAN'S HOSPITAL—North College Avenue and 22d Street. &
PENNSYLVANIA HOSPITAL—8th and Pine Streets.

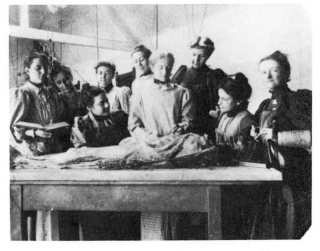

Left: *Class schedule, winter session, 1876–77.* ASCWM, MCP. Rights: *Students dissecting, Woman's Medical College of Pennsylvania (c. 1890).* ASCWM, MCP.

I am very busy, as you will imagine, when I tell you of eight courses of lectures . . . five clinics, [and] four quizzes . . . to attend in each week.
                                                                    –Harriet Belcher, 1876

Anatomy

I have not begun dissecting, as the material on hand did not present a very attractive appearance. I am waiting for cooler weather and until some unfortunate victim sees his way clear to devote his mortal remains to the advancement of science.
                                                                    –Rachel Nicol, 1876

From what I hear of other colleges, I have no doubt that dissection as managed by women is a very different matter from one taken under the charge of male attendants. Every precaution is taken to spare the senses.   –Harriet Belcher, 1875

Pharmacy

Among the specialties of the Spring Session may be mentioned a course in Practical Pharmacy. This is worthy of particular notice on account of the importance to physicians of being able to discriminate between preparations of competent and of incompetent druggists, whose field trenches so closely upon that of the prescriber. The familiarity with standard medicinal preparations which comes from actual manipulation in the laboratory, gives a confidence in judgment not to be secured in any other way.   –Annual Announcement, 1876

Clinical Experience

The 1876 Annual Announcement of the Woman's Medical College of Pennsylvania boasted, "Excellent clinical advantages are within reach of the stu-

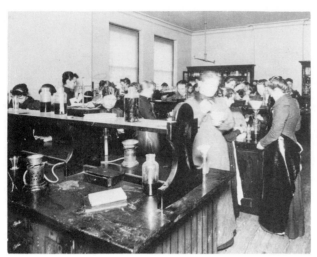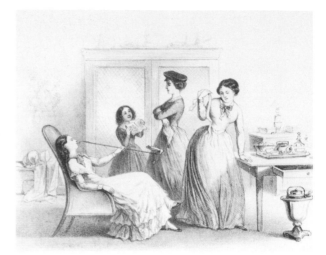

Left: *Pharmaceutical lab, Woman's Medical College of Pennsylvania, (c. 1890).* ASCWM, MCP. Right: *Drawing of women smoking opium.* Ann Abram Collection

dents of this college." Four different opportunities for practical study were open to the students.

The Woman's Medical College Dispensary, an outpatient service founded in 1858, and the Woman's Hospital of Philadelphia, founded in 1861, were typical of the experience offered within the woman's medical sphere.

In spite of their success in establishing women's medical institutions, nineteenth-century women doctors continued to press for the right to attend male medical institutions. By 1876, students from the Woman's Medical College could attend coeducational clinical lectures at both the Philadelphia Hospital (Almshouse) and the Pennsylvania Hospital.

Dispensary

The Woman's Hospital, where over four thousand patients are treated annually, is in the immediate neighborhood of the College. Its daily dispensary service is open to the students, under proper restrictions. –Annual Announcement, 1876

I went to Front Street about 4 A.M. and had a forceps case about 8 A.M. . . . After church, went to see a woman who had taken too much opium. . . . Saw five drunken women. –Anna Kugler, 1877

Bedside instruction is given daily to a limited number by the resident physician, Anna E. Broomal, M.D. –Annual Announcement, 1876

Weekly Clinics

Weekly Clinics in the various departments are held by the different members of the attending staff. The cases presented at these clinics being supplied by the wards of the hospital, and from its dispensary service, represent those classes of diseases which

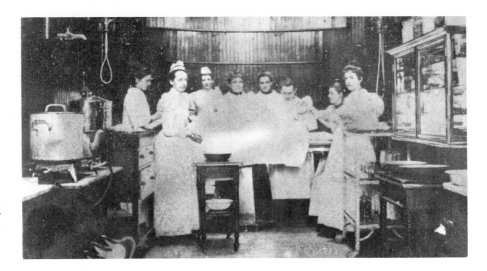

Students attending operation, Woman's Hospital, Philadelphia (c. 1885), ASCWM, MCP.

the graduates will most frequently be called upon to treat; hence these clinics are peculiarly valuable. —Annual Announcement, 1876

The clinics are what try my soul. . . . It needs all the resolution I am mistress of to not be overwhelmed with horror and pity for the poor unfortunates who are compelled by their poverty to subject themselves to what must seem to them a cruel and unsympathetic curiosity. I thought I . . . realized what I had to encounter, but I never really imagined such horrors of disease and deformity as I have seen.
—Harriet Belcher, 1875

"Mixed" Clinics

Although the Woman's Medical College was proud to be able to offer access to coeducational clinical training to its students, some found it difficult to adjust outside the separate sphere.

The most absurd of all things is coming away here to attend a woman's medical college and then to attend clinics with five or six tallow-brained, dough-faced specimens of the genus homo. I fail to see [how] . . . a hundred would be worse than five. —Rachel Nicol, 1876

The hardest thing I have had to face since I began have been the mixed clinics. The authorities have consented to admit women to the clinics at Blockley Almshouse, a very great advantage. —Harriet Belcher, 1878

Amusement

Life at the Woman's Medical College was not without its social pleasures. In 1876, responding to a request from the students, the college suspended classes, allowing the ladies an opportunity to attend the Great Centennial Exhibition in Philadelphia. There, in the Women's pavilion, a pharmaceutical display by the Woman's Medical College was very well received.

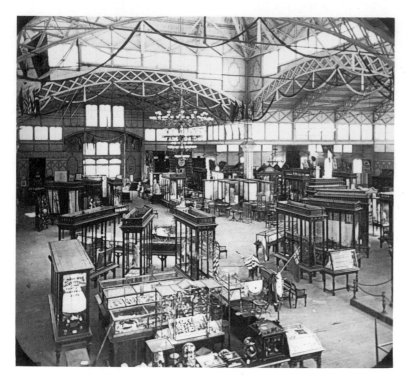

The Woman's Pavilion, 1876 Centennial, Philadelphia. National Archives.

A request by the students for a holiday on Election Day, Tuesday, November 7, which was Woman's Day at the Centennial Exhibition was granted so they could go. —Minutes of the Woman's Medical College of Pennsylvania, 1876.

I went out yesterday afternoon with three others to pack up our exhibit, and We had made our plans to keep at work till about 8 P.M. totally unaware that all doors were closed at five. It was exasperating to contemplate undoing all our afternoon's work and locking them up in the cases again. [Finally] two of us took the large and each of the others two small baskets and marched past those objecting guards. . . .
—Harriet Belcher, 1876

More everyday pleasures of student life included the camaraderie of sister students in the boarding houses near the college.

Of no small importance to me is that I have a very pleasant home-like boarding house, I am not the only boarder. Nothing could be plainer than the furniture and appointments, but everything is as neat as wax, and the people, who are Quakers, are as kind and pleasant as possible. —Harriet Belcher, 1875

Examinations

A final examination and a thesis were the last hurdles to be overcome before the degree of M.D. could be conferred.

We poor mortals are shaking in our shoes at the prospect of the examinations. Did

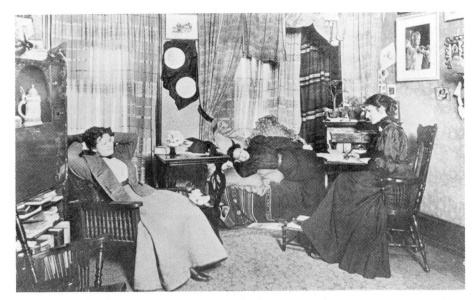

Students from the Woman's Medical College of Pennsylvania relaxing in boarding house room near college (c. 1890). ASCWM, MCP. *(Original caption from Daughters of Aesculapius,* Woman's Medical College of Pennsylvania.

I ever tell you of what use our old studies of Latin and even the smattering of Greek have been to me . . . ?   –Harriet Belcher, 1877

In the months prior to exams, tension ran high. Students turned to each other for help and support.

I have agreed to quiz one of my fellow-students on physiology and shall have to study like a Trojan for it lest she may find out that she knows as much or more about it than I do. . . . Another one wanted me to take her on chemistry but that was too much for she, poor soul, is mortally stupid and it would have tired me out for nothing. . . .   –Harriet Belcher, 1876

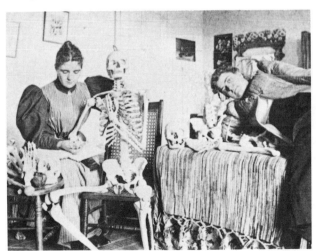
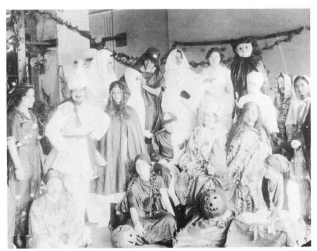

Left: *Three and a half friends from the Woman's Medical College of Pennsylvania in boarding house room (c. 1895).* ASCWM, MCP. Right: *Students' Halloween party, Woman's Medical College of Pennsylvania (c. 1898).* ASCWM, MCP.

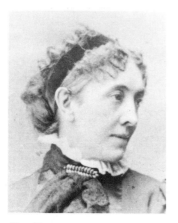

Dr. Frances Emily White, Professor of Physiology, Woman's Medical College of Pennsylvania, 1877–1904. ASCWM, MCP.

Student protest was not invented in the 1960s. Charging that they were inadequately prepared in physiology, forty students petitioned for removal of a professor.

We the undersigned students respectfully state to the Board of Corporators that we wish to return to this college to complete our course but feel that the lectures on physiology have been wholly inadequate to our needs as students and in our future work. We therefore beg most earnestly that the present incumbent of that chair be removed. —Petition to the Board of Corporators, 1877

The faculty voted to "sustain Professor White in the position which she has taken with regard to the discourtesy shown her by a portion of the class during her lecture hour." However, at the end of the year, and over the objection of Professor White and Professor Clara Marshall, the faculty eased the pass requirement in view "of the distracting influences which have existed during the present session" (—Minutes of the Faculty of the Woman's Medical College of Pennsylvania, 1876).

After examinations, the professors met to grade the students by rolling balls. White balls represented plus points; black balls, minus.

Thesis

[Candidate for the M.D. degree must] present . . . a thesis for her own penmanship, on some subject which has direct application to medicine.
—Annual Announcement, 1876–77.

And not the least of my woes is the horrid thesis, which has been my bête noir ever since I began to study. —Harriet Belcher, 1878.

THESIS TOPICS OF THE CLASS OF 1879

Mary Alice Avery, *The Bath*
Emma A. Baldwin, *Food*
Harriet G. Belcher, *Drainage*
Sarah Alice Cohen, *Syphilis*
Martha M. Dunn, *Internal Diseases of Women*
Henrietta Louisa Exton, *Disinfection*
Phoebe H. Flagler, *Scarlatina*
Eleanor E. Galt, *Absorption of Fat*
Sophia E. Howard, *The Hand*
Agnes Nininger Kemp, *Pyrolapsi Uteri*
Anna S. Kugler, *Acute Bright's Disease*
Rachel J. Nicol, *Cholera Infantum*
Julia P. Pease, *Alcohol as Food*
Sophia Presley, *Acquired Syphilis*
Almina F. Rhodes, *The Physician's Duty as Educator*
Ida E. Richardson, *Eczema*

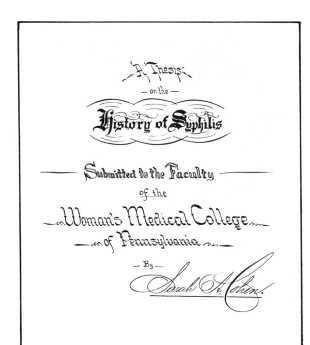

Title page of Sarah Cohen's senior thesis, Woman's Medical College of Pennsylvania, 1879. ASCWM, MCP.

Louise Schneider, *Aenesthesia in Natural Labor*
Lucy R. Weaver, *Puerperal Peronitis*
Mary H. Wolfenden, *Toenia Solium*
Mina Fitch Wood, *Entero-Colitus Infantum*

Excerpts from senior theses reveal the students' knowledge of the standard therapeutics of their day. Harriet Belcher's concern with preventive medicine was in keeping with the progressive Woman's Medical College, where the subject would one day warrant a class of its own.

Causes of Idropathic Eczema: "Chemical Irritants, high temperatures, low temperatures, excessive perspiration, prolonged prickly heat, sudden changes in the weather."
–Ida Richardson, *Exzema*

"[Syphilis is transmitted by] impure intercourse [indulged in by] men and women who . . . disregard the laws of God and Man." –Sophia Presley, *Acquired Syphilis*

"Cold [is the] chief cause of [inflammation of the kidneys] in adults."
–Anna Kugler, *Acute Bright's Disease*

"[There is a debate] over the manner in which infection is conveyed from one being to another." –Henrietta Exton, *Disinfection*

"The derangement of one tissue in some degree affects all."
–Emma Baldwin, *The Therapeutics of Food*

GIVE HER KNOWLEDGE

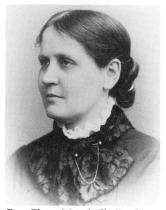

Dr. Clara Marshall, Professor of Materia Medica and Therapeutics, Woman's Medical College of Pennsylvania, 1876–1905 (1880s). ASCWM, MCP.

"There is a tendency among some physicians to attribute many diseases to microscopic spores, fungi, or animalculae. There may be some reason for this [but] it is by no means certain whether they are the cause. . . . There is no proof of belladonna's effectiveness [in the treatment of scarlatina] but it is harmless and friends often wish it."
—Phoebe Flagler, *On Scarlatina*

"Preventive medicine will be regarded as the most important department in the curriculum of science. . . . [The physician is] admitted to all homes in the most confidential relations, [giving him] a heavy obligation to use that influence in all directions for the best service of humanity. . . . [The medical profession is] best fitted to comprehend the subject [of sanitation and therefore most responsible for] influencing the community at large."
—Harriet Belcher, *Sanitary Drainage*

Graduation

I wish you could happen along on March 13th. Would like to see you on my wedding day.
—Harriet Belcher, 1879.

And finally, on March 13, 1879, graduation day arrived. Dressed in pristine white dresses, the twenty graduates of the twenty-ninth class of the Woman's Medical College of Pennsylvania heard Dr. Clara Marshall, professor of Ma-

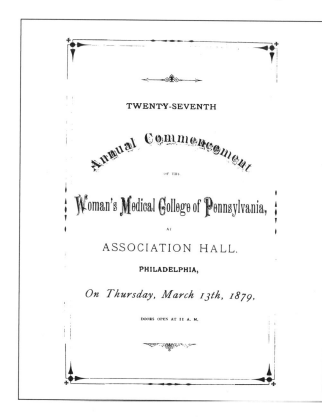

TWENTY-SEVENTH

Annual Commencement

OF THE

Woman's Medical College of Pennsylvania,

AT

ASSOCIATION HALL.

PHILADELPHIA,

On Thursday, March 13th, 1879,

DOORS OPEN AT 11 A. M.

COMMENCEMENT.

The Twenty-Seventh Annual Commencement was held at Association Hall, Philadelphia, on Thursday, March 13th, 1879, at 12 M., when the Degree of Doctor of Medicine was conferred by the President, T. Morris Perot, Esq., upon the following named ladies:

NAMES.	RESIDENCE.	SUBJECT OF THESIS.
M. ALICE AVERY,	New Hampshire,	The Physiological Action of Baths.
EMMA A. BALDWIN,	Illinois,	Therapeutics of Food.
HARRIET G. BELCHER,	New Jersey,	Sanitary Drainage.
SARAH A. COHEN,	Pennsylvania,	History of Syphilis.
MARTHA M. DUNN,	New York,	Intestinal Diseases of Children.
H. LOUISA EXTON,	New Jersey,	Disinfection.
PHEBE H. FLAGLER,	Pennsylvania,	Scarlatina.
ELEANOR E. GALT,	New York,	Absorption of Fats.
SOPHIA E. HOWARD,	New York,	The Hand.
AGNES KEMP,	Pennsylvania,	Prolapsus Uteri.
ANNA S. KUGLER,	Pennsylvania,	Acute Bright's Disease.
RACHEL J. NICOL,	Illinois,	Cholera Infantum.
JULIA P. PEASE,	Vermont,	Alcohol as a Food.
SOPHIA PRESLEY,	Ohio,	Acquired Syphilis.
IDA E. RICHARDSON,	Pennsylvania.	Eczema.
ALMINA F. RHODES,	Pennsylvania,	The Physician's Duty as an Educator.
LOUISE SCHNEIDER,	Pennsylvania.	Anæsthesia in Natural Labor.
LUCY R. WEAVER,	Rhode Island.	Symptoms of Puerperal Peritonitis.
MINA FITCH WOOD,	New York.	Entero-Colitis of Infancy.
MARY H. WOLFENDEN,	Massachusetts.	Tænia Solium.

The Honorary Degree of Doctor of Medicine was conferred by the President upon Prof. Rachel L. Bodley, A.M., of Philadelphia.

The Valedictory Address to the Graduates was delivered by Clara Marshall, M. D., Professor of Materia Medica and General Therapeutics.

Program for the Twenty-seventh Annual Commencement, Woman's Medical College of Pennsylvania. ASCWM, MCP.

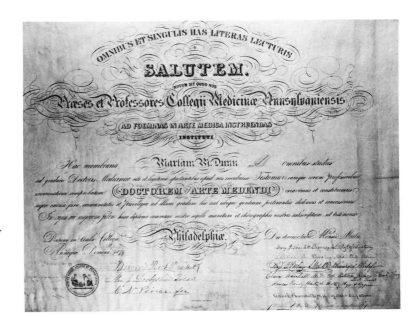

Diploma of Dr. Martha M. Dunn, Woman's Medical College of Pennsylvania, 1879. Corey Family Collection.

teria Medica, deliver the commencement address "in a prose most clear."

"Care for your knowledge as you would a tender plant," Dr. Marshall cautioned the graduates; "Let no blighting frost of unsympathizing companionship kill it before it becomes strong." Reminding the graduates of the valiant efforts by earlier pioneers to open the doors of medicine to women, Dr. Marshall urged the new physicians to "seek and take advantage of opportunities; despise no opening wedge, however small. Be baffled in no rightful undertaking, however formidable. Every improved circumstance comes as a helping hand, not only to the profession, but to our sex." She reminded the graduates of the barriers still to overcome: "[Women physicians] still carry the burden of a two-fold responsibility: fidelity to a great cause and devotion to the interests of a noble profession." Dr. Marshall took advantage of this last appearance before the whole class to discuss the nature of their relationship with their future patients, counseling, "The family physician frequently becomes the valued friend of the family. You bar yourselves from the use of a valuable instrument when you refuse to study people as well as diseases. You will often reach patients and cure them too, by a scientific use of your humanity." Never one to mince words, Dr. Marshall declared, "The woman of society is too often its slave. You should be wise enough and shrewd enough to make society serve you."

With their leader's words ringing in their ears, the members of the twenty-ninth graduating class stepped out into the world . . . as physicians.

Postgraduate Training

After graduation, three of the students sailed to Europe for postgraduate education. Rachel Nicol and Louise Schneider (Blum) went to Zurich. Martha

Dunn (Corey) practiced for six years and then left for England to study with the famed surgeon and antivivisectionist, Dr. Lawson Tait.

Not one to take his preceptor responsibilities lightly, Dr. Tait sent Dr. Dunn regular announcements of his upcoming operations so she could attend; he followed her career long after she had returned to the United States.

NOTES

1. First Annual Announcement, Female Medical College of Pennsylvania, 1850 (Philadelphia: Archives and Special Collections on Women in Medicine, Medical College of Pennsylvania).
2. Sarah A. Dolley, "Closing Lecture to the Class of 1879" (Philadelphia: Archives and Special Collections on Women in Medicine, Medical College of Pennsylvania).

Private Practice

Taking Every Case to Heart

RUTH J. ABRAM

166 are now engaged in active practice. Gynaecological and obstetrical practice predominates. The average income is $2,907.30. Four Report from $15,000 to $20,000.
                                                    –Dr. Rachel Bodley, Dean
Survey of the Living Graduates of the Woman's
Medical College of Pennsylvania, 1881

Type of Practice: Alumnae, Woman's Medical College of Pennsylvania

32: gynecological
10: obstetrical
10: medical
 3: surgical
37: general practice
23: gynecological and obstetrical
 6: gynecological and surgical
29: gynecological and medical
 9: obstetrical and medical
 7: surgical and medical

153

Private Practice

Mary Alice Avery: Portland, Maine

Emma Baldwin: Chicago, Illinois

Harriet G. Belcher: Pawtucket, Rhode Island
       Santa Barbara, California

Sarah Alice Cohen May: Philadelphia, Pennsylvania

Martha Dunn Corey: Utica, New York
      Waterbury, Connecticut
      Pacific Beach, California
      Marion, Ohio
      Springfield, Ohio
      La Jolla, California

Henrietta Lousia Exton: Union Township, New Jersey

Phoebe Flagler Hagenbuch: Strousburg, Pennsylvania
        Bryan, Ohio
        Williamsport, Pennsylvania
        Stroudsburg, Pennsylvania

Eleanor Galt Simmons: Courtland, New York
       Philadelphia, Pennsylvania
       Elizabeth, New Jersey
       New York, New York
       Coconut Grove, Florida

Sophia E. Howard: Auburn, New York
      Fairport, New York

Agnes Nininger Kemp: Harrisburg, Pennsylvania

Julia Pease Abbott: Rutland, Vermont

Sophia Presley: Camden, New Jersey

Almina Rhodes Dean: Cambridgeboro, Pennsylvania

Louise Schneider Blum: Philadelphia, Pennsylvania
       York, Pennsylvania

Lucy Rhodes Weaver: Pawtucket, Rhode Island

Mary Wolfenden Battershall: Attleboro, Massachusett

Mina Fitch Wood: Cortland, New York

In his best-selling advice book for physicians, Dr. D. W. Cathell advised beginning practitioners to "hesitate to take such offices as vaccine physician, coroner, city dispensary physician, santiary inspector, etc.," explaining that such affiliations "usually create a low grade reputation that it is hard to outlive." If the physician had "any merit at all," said Cathell, he should pursue a private practice.[1]

Women physicians practicing in the late nineteenth century were not burdened by quite the same suspicion attending their male colleagues. The Victorian concept of "Virtuous Womanhood," which ascribed heightened moral sensibilities to women, protected them. Most members of the Class of 1879 accepted positions in institutions. They viewed it as an extension of their training and also as a means of fulfilling their special mission as social healers. At the same time, most of them viewed their institutional practices as a step toward their ultimate goal, establishing a private practice. For them, as for most nineteenth-century physicians, the preferred practice was a private one, based at home, with a middle-class clientele. The fact that most nineteenth-century physicians practiced from their homes was a particular aid to women physicians. For those with family responsibilities, it offered more flexibility. It also permitted them to stay within the bounds of society's view that woman's place was at home. And when they left home, it was for the "purpose of making home enjoyments more complete . . . [and] to bear health and hope to the abodes [they] enter."[2]

Dr. Cathell offered tips on how to attract this desired middle-class clientele. A primary consideration was competition. The choice of the right location was key. It was "risky for a beginner," wrote Cathell, "to locate in a section already overstocked with popular, energetic physicians."[3]

No doubt familiar with Cathell's work, Dr. Harriet Belcher reviewed her options. She was, she wrote, "strongly advised by several people to settle in Burlington, Vermont, where there is no lady physician."[4] Women physicians depended upon a female clientele who, out of either feminist conviction or Victorian modesty—or both, sought out women doctors. There was, therefore, an ironic advantage to being a woman physician in 1880. When listing themselves in city directories, female physicians routinely distinguished themselves from their male colleagues by using their full names rather than first initials, lest anyone looking for a female physician pass them over.

Although in their public utterances Victorian women physicians often assured their male colleagues that they represented no competition since they treated women who would endure pain and even death rather than visit male physicians, the truth was that female patients provided the opening wedge into a general practice. Reminiscing about his grandmother, Dr. Phoebe Flagler Hagenbuch, William Hoffman said: "I have heard stories of table top operations. . . . One man in the neighborhood . . . had his arm amputated under these conditions by her. He had gotten it caught in a corn shucker."[5] Dr. Sarah Cohen May's neighbor remembered that the doctor had treated her father for asthma.[6] Invoices of Phoebe Flagler Hagenbuch and Almina Rhodes Dean clearly show that their practices were not limited to women and children. Perhaps the *Miami Metropolis*'s account of one of Dr. Eleanor Galt Simmons's patients provides the most dramatic evidence of this point. Simmons was called to treat a man mortally wounded by a bandit in Miami. After dressing his wounds, Simmons "offered to help [the bandit]" who was "holed up in a shack after killing two men in broad day light." The bandit accepted Simmons's offer "on condition that the lady doctor come unarmed. She removed three bullets from his thighs, dressed his wounds, and splinted the compound fracture of his leg. She refused his request for enough chloroform to kill him."[7]

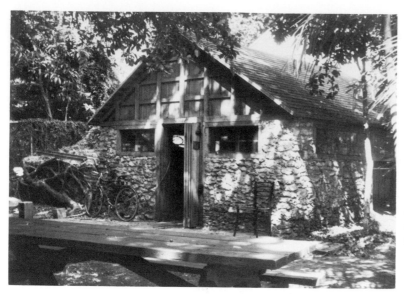

Office of Eleanor Galt Simmons, Coconut Grove, Florida. Gertrude M. Kent Collection.

While women physicians usually had a preponderance of female and child patients, they did not advertise themselves as specialists, lest they narrow their patient appeal.

A new physician required introductions to the "right" people in town. It was the promise of such introductions that finally decided Harriet Belcher to settle in Pawtucket, Rhode Island. Pawtucket was the home of Harriet's roommate, Dr. Lucy Weaver, who, with her preceptor, Dr. Anita Tyng, promised "introductions social and professional and all the help [they] could give." Furthermore, Harriet wrote a friend, Dr. Tyng, "has a good practice in Providence and a number of patients in Pawtucket whom she is anxious to hand over to someone else."[8] Harriet clearly hoped to be that "someone else."

Members of the Class of 1879 made the necessary connections in a number of ways. Mary Alice Avery accepted the offer of her preceptor, Dr. Elizabeth Keller, to join her private Boston practice. Avery was surely pleased, for Dr. Keller was an accomplished surgeon, former physician to the New England Hospital for Women and Children in Boston, and daughter of a well-to-do New England family.

Older, more established classmates lent a hand as well. Dr. Martha Dunn went to work with Dr. Charlotte Merrick, who had a burgeoning practice in Utica, New York.[9] The daughter of prominent Canadians, Dr. Merrick had graduated the year before from the Woman's Medical College of Pennsylvania.

In this tendency to affiliate, nineteenth-century women physicians again breached one of Dr. Cathell's precepts. "Contact no entangling alliances," he advised. "It is better not to enter into partnerships with other physicians. . . . The sooner you learn to depend wholly on yourself the better."[10] But evidence was everywhere for women physicians that *only* by forming alliances would they prosper. Their leadership urged them to help one another, and they did.

Another way to ensure oneself the necessary connections was to return home. This was the solution for most of those who elected private practices (and all except one eventually did). For Henrietta Lousia Exton, connections in Hunterdon County were the least of her worries. Her family *was* Hunterdon County. Nor were finances a problem, so Exton was free to pursue her passionate interest in the antivivisection and vegetarian movements. (In her will, Dr. Exton bequeathed money to both the American Anti-vivisecture Society and the American Society for the Prevention of Cruelty to Animals. She also left money for the maintenance of her pet sheep.) For Phoebe Flagler Hagenbuch, Stroudsburg provided a welcoming atmosphere. An integral member of the town's Quaker community, Dr. Hagenbuch had little reason to fear professional starvation. Almina Rhodes Dean was similarly fortunate. Her family's farm, financial backing, and community standing offered the support she needed. Upon returning home, Almina and her mother established a small invalid home.

Sarah Cohen May had a different set of problems when she commenced her practice. At twenty-one, she was, as she would later boast, the youngest member of her class.[11] The daughter of poor, Orthodox Jewish immigrants, Sarah was also the least well connected. After her father's death following the failure of his watch repairing business during the Depression of 1873, Sarah lived with her brothers and depressed mother on Philadelphia's immigrant South Side.

In spite of her difficulties, Sarah did have a peculiar advantage, and she used it right away. In 1879, she was the only Jewish woman physician in the

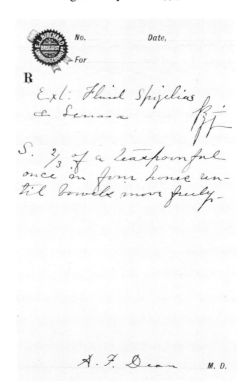

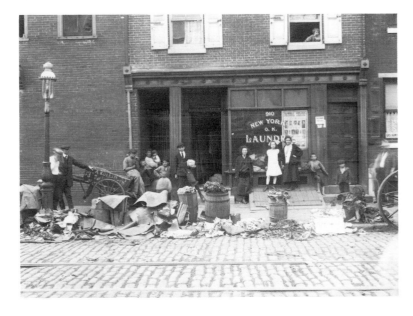

Left: *Prescription from Dr. Almina Rhodes Dean (1880s).* Kreitz Family Collection. Right above: *Home of Dr. Almina Rhodes Dean, Cambridge Springs, Pennsylvania.* Kreitz Family Collection.

city. At a time when western European Jews were fleeing to the United States (and to Philadelphia) in record numbers, Sarah Cohen May was available. She established her practice among these immigrants. Sarah knew the birthing rituals, the social decorum between women and men, and she knew the language. Her delivery records, filed with the city's Department of Health, tell the story clearly. Between February and June, 1880, Sarah reported the following cases:

2/3 Abrahama and Esther Miller, 831 Christian Street, Watchmaker
2/10 Wolf and Jennie Razovskie, 316 Lock Street, Peddler
3/13 Jacob and Caroline Marluk, 605 Poplar St., Merchant
3/14 Joseph and Elizabeth Emanuel, 662 Vane St., Peddler
3/28 Simon and Ida Nathans, 857 No. 8th St., Merchant
5/2 Abraham and Celia Weinbach, 1244 Mervine St., Clerk
6/22 Asher and Gertrude Michael, 612 Wayne St., Tailor
6/27 Simon and Sarah Wessell, 2636 Lock St., Peddler[12]

The watchmakers, peddlers, merchants, clerks, tailors, shoemakers, and in November of that year, the rabbi's wife, became Sarah's connection with the middle-class life for which she yearned.[13] After delivery, the family would require a physician for the baby, and then, while she was at it, could something be done for the husband's cough? Dr. Sarah Cohen May was on her way to a thriving family practice. She was joined, in 1881, by her elder brother, Morris, a graduate of Jefferson Medical College, and their younger brother, Isaac, a graduate of the Philadelphia College of Pharmacy. This joint venture lasted seven years until the brothers married.

Harriet Belcher had no intention of stepping over filth to find her way to the back rooms of city tenements. From the beginning, she angled for a middle-class, if not upper-class, practice. Her faith in the importance of social introductions was not misplaced. It was on account of them, she wrote just months after arriving in Pawtucket, that she had "not had a disagreeable experience of any kind." The Episcopal pastor had paid a courtesy call. Even the cashier at the local bank promised to do all he could "to get me into practice, for he wanted me to stay."[14]

A newly coined physician had to take care in selecting the proper neighborhood in which to locate. According to Dr. Cathell, the physician should select "a congenial . . . place . . . in a genteel neighborhood . . . upon or very near an artery of travel. . . ." A corner house was best because an office entrance could be constructed on a side street and the additional light aided "examinations, operations, and study."[15] Harriet Belcher settled the matter with her usual efficiency and attention to detail, renting space in a pleasant neighborhood in which "most of the houses are large and with grounds around them." Then she went to work fixing up her rooms, reporting the particulars to her friend:

The office is about 8 by 12 feet, is prettily carpeted and papered, and has lounge, wardrobe, office chair, and large desk of stained wood. [The landlady] added a grand old mirror . . . and a table to do duty as washstand, which, with the lounge, I have covered with very pretty chintz. . . . A pretty towel rack which I have filled in with English Embroidery, my diploma, books, etc. are all that I have had to add, except for the windows. I have had a black curtain bar with gold knobs and rings put up at the ceiling and have made handings of burlap with bands of maroon velveteen catstitched on with gold color. [They] give quite an 'air' to the establishment.[16]

Despite the introductions, invitations, and her lovely office, it was a month before Harriet's first patient arrived. It was a "young girl who imagined she had cancer. The purest fancy, as I told her. I was then called to attend an old lady who has injured her eye so severely that I [may] have to take her to a specialist. She can only pay me in gratitude."[17]

Harriet's concern over her dearth of patients was temporarily forgotten during her first winter when she was absorbed in "studying carefully and preparing for an operation" at which she was to assist Dr. Tyng. The date was set for January 8.

Five physicians, all women, opened the abdomen and removed two small ovarian tumors and one of another kind. . . . Then for three weeks, I remained and took care of [the patient] night and day. I can't tell you what a mental and physical strain the first few days were, nor the utter thankfulness with which we saw her coming through safely. . . . Success or failure was so much more to us professionally than it would have been to men.[18]

By midsummer, however, Harriet's distress was pronounced. Writing her friend Eliza Johnson, the physician admitted:

I am mercenary as possible and growing no better fast. I am beginning to look at everyone with a single eye as to how much, in cash, they are good for. And the sick ones get well so disgustingly fast that I want to poison them mildly, just to keep them hanging on my hands. And the poor ones have such hard time in the struggle for existence, I can't make it any harder, so I charge them very little.[19]

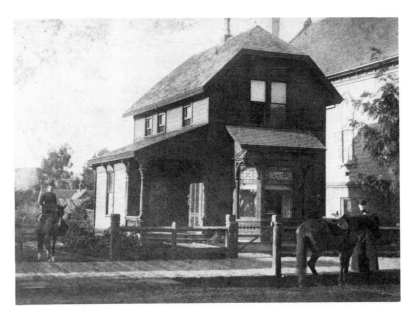

Dr. Harriet Belcher standing beside her horse in front of her office on State Street in Santa Barbara, California (c. 1882). Santa Barbara Historical Society.

After two years, Harriet decided to relocate to the winter resort town of Santa Barbara. There, her fortunes rose. In her first month, she reported "more business than I ever had in Rhode Island." Two papers, Harriet wrote, greeted her arrival enthusiastically when "I inserted my card": "Miss Belcher, our new resident physician, is swiftly and surely winning the hearts and confidence of the ladies. . . . Her success and popularity are unquestioned."[20]

Harriet was under no illusions as to the reason for the enthusiasm, telling her friend that "the secret of this little puff" was that the "Editress came to me . . . suffering . . . from an attack of piles." Apparently, Harriet's prescription "worked like a charm."[21]

It was customary for nineteenth-century physicians to advertise their availability in the local newspaper. The *Courtland Standard*, in Courtland, New York, often carried information supplied by Dr. Mina Fitch Wood:

Dr. Mina F. Wood has recovered from her illness and has returned from New York where for the past six weeks she has been attending lectures and making particular study of microscopy and doing other special work. She will reopen her office . . . next week where she may be found until 9 o'clock in the morning and from two to 5 o'clock in the afternoon and from 7 to 9 o'clock in the evening.[22]

Harriet Belcher's practice expanded rapidly. Her office hours were typical: 10 to 12 and 2 to 4. But, as she reported, she was generally in her office until 8 P.M.[23]

Harriet's practice supplied the downpayment for a house, "one of the prettiest in town. Under the bay window in front is a mass of lobelia. . . . A scarlet passion vine runs riot over the trellis and the roses are already blooming."[24]

In the summer of 1885, the doctor "took off a breast for cancer, though two other physicians had not considered that disease." It was also the summer she contended with "the worst case of hysteria" she had ever seen "and fifteen miles out in the country": a homeopathic physician asked her "to take a case of puerperal insanity off his hands."[25]

Harriet Belcher's hectic schedule caused her to opine that she was "glad on the whole [that she had] a small practice, I think I shall never break myself of taking every case to heart."[26]

The variety of Harriet's practice was not unusual for nineteenth-century physicians. Indeed, in his discussion of physician's office signs, Dr. Cathell advised them not to add " 'Physician and Surgeon' or 'Physician and Accoucheur' " as "all physicians are supposed to be surgeons, accoucheurs, etc. . . . The medical case of today is the surgical or obstetrical case of tomorrow. . . ."[27]

And every case called upon the physician's pharmaceutical skills. Although a physician who compounded his own drugs risked the ire of the town's pharmacists, many chose to do so. Phoebe Flagler Hagenbuch's grandson remembered his grandmother's routine request of her adopted son, "Willie, I would like thee to take me to the fields tomorrow." There Phoebe would collect the ferns, roots, and other wild materials for her medicine. "She used some combination of roots and leaves from three different plants, well boiled together, cooled and strained, to treat my poison ivy." William Hoffman

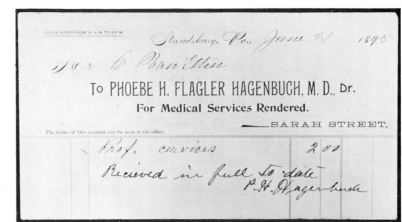

Dr. Hagenbuch's receipt for payment (1895).
Monroe County Historical Society.

swears it was the best remedy he has ever had for the affliction. "She used spider webs to stop a cut from bleeding. Her pharmacy had shelf after shelf of apothacary jars filled with all sorts of good smelling powders, roots and herbs."[28]

Victorian women physicians hoped to support themselves and their families through their work. As early as 1858, Dr. Ann Preston, dean of the Woman's Medical College of Pennsylvania, had explained that it was hoped that the practice of medicine would "be a means of pecuniary independence."[29] Dean Rachel Bodley's survey confirmed that in this regard, women physicians were meeting with success. Certainly, members of the Class of 1879 did. Their assets at the time of their deaths averaged over eighteen thousand dollars. Some, such as Henrietta Exton, undoubtedly owed much of their well-being to inheritance. But she was the exception to the rule. Dr. Martha Dunn Corey, orphaned at an early age and sent to live with an impoverished preacher, was abandoned by her husband after the birth of her third child. She deserves

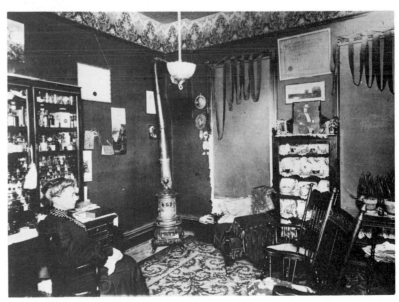

Dr. Mary Bishop posing in her office
(c. 1898). Burns Archive.

full credit for amassing an estate worth over eighty thousand dollars. When Harriet Belcher died prematurely at the age of forty-five, one of her friends wrote Belcher's relative saying that her practice "had got to be a fine one. There was no one in town who was so loved and who will be missed by so many. She died a happy woman, well assured of her success in life."[30]

Similar expressions of the important regard in which communities held members of the Class of 1879, and all late-nineteenth-century women physicians, were forthcoming at the time of their deaths. Dr. Mary Alice Avery's colleagues in Portland, Maine, memorialized her, calling her "wise, courageous, and untiring . . . a skillful obstetrician and gynecologist. In the understanding and treatment of . . . little children, she had no superior. Her face itself was a wonderful power."[31]

NOTES

1. D. W. Cathell, M.D., *The Physician Himself and Things That Concern His Reputation and Success*, 9th ed. (Philadelphia: F. A. Davis, 1890), 20.
2. Ann Preston, M.D., "Valedictory Address, Female Medical College of Pennsylvania," 1858.
3. Cathell, *The Physician Himself,* 4.
4. Harriet Belcher to Eliza Johnson, August 10, 1878. All letters from Belcher to Johnson referred to in this essay are from the Alice McCone Collection.
5. William Hoffman, letter to author.
6. Elizabeth Stern, interview with author.
7. *Miami Metropolis,* July 2, 1909.
8. Harriet Belcher to Eliza Johnson, February 5, 1879. Alice McCone Collection.
9. Obituary of Charlotte Merrick, *Utica Morning Herald,* March 20, 1899.
10. Cathell, *The Physician Himself,* 2.
11. Elizabeth Stern interview.
12. Birth Records, City Archives, Philadelphia.
13. Diary of Rabbi Elias Eppstein.
14. Harriet Belcher to Eliza Johnson, July 13, 1879.
15. Cathell, *The Physician Himself,* 5.
16. Harriet Blecher to Eliza Johnson, July 13, 1879.
17. Harriet Belcher to Eliza Johnson, November 16, 1879.
18. Harriet Belcher to Eliza Johnson, February 9, 1880.
19. Harriet Belcher to Eliza Johnson, July 11, 1880.
20. Harriet Belcher to Eliza Johnson, February 6, 1882.
21. Ibid.
22. *Courtland Standard.* January 7, 1886.
23. Harriet Belcher to Eliza Johnson, October 4, 1885.
24. Ibid.
25. Ibid.
26. Ibid.
27. Cathell, *The Physician Himself,* 11.
28. William Hoffman, letter to author.
29. Ann Preston, M.D. "Valedictory Address," Female Medical College of Pennsylvania, 1858.
30. Rebecca S. Moor to Eliza Johnson, June 12, 1887.
31. Portland Newspaper, name and date unknown. Women's Medical College of Pennsylvania Scrapbook Collection, ACC no. 133: 323. Archives and Special Collections on Women in Medicine, Medical College of Pennsylvania.

Teaching

"For Which Woman is Preeminently Fitted"

ELLEN J. SMITH

Question sixth referred to the work for which woman is preeminently fitted, that of medical teacher, and specified separately institutions of learning, and popular audiences of women. Fifty-five [of 189 respondents] answer this question affirmatively.
—Dr. Rachel Bodley, Dean
Survey of the Living Graduates of the Woman's
Medical College of Pennsylvania, 1881

Members of the Class of 1879 Who Taught

Belcher: Lecturer before women's groups
Cohen (May): Anatomy demonstrator, Philadelphia College of Osteopathy
Exton: Writer on vegetarianism
Galt (Simmons): Lecturer before women's groups
Howard: Lecturer before women's and children's groups
Kemp: Lecturer before women's and temperance groups
Kugler: Professor at the Women's Medical College of Pennsylvania and at
    her mission hospital in Guntur, India
Presley: Professor at the Woman's Medical College of Pennsylvania and at
    the New Jersey Training School for Nurses, Camden
Richardson: Professor at the Woman's Medical College of Pennsylvania

163

Weaver (Soule): Lecturer before women's groups
Wolfenden (Battershall): Lecturer before women's groups

The fact that nineteenth-century women physicians succeeded as well as they did in private practice and institutional work resulted directly from the quality of training they received in medical school and in their postgraduate training. Generally barred from attending male medical schools and internship programs in affiliated hospitals, nineteenth-century female medical students enrolled in women's medical colleges and clinical programs, where they were trained primarily by women physicians. The new graduates, in their turn, became part of the group of women qualified to educate and train future women doctors, both as their instructors in medical schools and as their preceptors and partners in postgraduate training and private practice. The reliance of women physicians on their own sex to train and educate them made teaching an essential aspect of the work of nineteenth-century women physicians.

Nor was the role of medical women as teachers confined to medical and nursing schools. Victorian ideology defined women as natural teachers and molders of society, particularly through their work in families. Women's abilities as educators included the capacity to shape moral and human character, to turn others toward improved ways of living, as well as simply to impart information. Nineteenth-century women doctors thus constantly placed themselves before general and popular audiences, bringing their messages of preventive medicine, public health, temperance sanitation, and basic data on physiology, health, and disease before the widest possible audience. With lecturing and teaching came active publishing careers, especially in popularly targeted pamphlets and articles. In educating future physicians, and the clientele they would eventually serve, nineteenth-century women doctors were serving the expectations of themselves both as Victorian women and as scientists and clinicians. Teaching was, as Dean Rachel Bodley of the Woman's Medical College of Pennsylvania put it, "work for which woman is preeminently fitted."[1] It was work in which nineteenth-century medical women entered in almost universal numbers.

"Medical teacher [in] institutions of higher learning . . ."

Women's medical colleges, and later, nursing schools, provided the institutional setting in which most women physicians pursued their formal teaching careers. Over the course of the nineteenth century, nineteen women's medical colleges were founded, and most of them sported predominantly female faculties. The Woman's Medical College of Pennsylvania, for example, began in 1850 with an all-male faculty of six professors. By 1876, enough women physicians had been trained there to support a faculty of nine women professors.[2] They taught all fields of the medical curriculum, from anatomy and dissecting to physiology to chemistry and material medica. In addition, they added a new curriculum to standard nineteenth-century training that reflected the women's medical movement's emphasis on public health and the health of women and children. Among the sections in the final examination given

Examination Questions.

SENIOR CLASS.

1. Lesions, primary and secondary, of cirrhosis of liver.
2. Symptoms of acute gastritis.
3. Treatment of acute Bright's disease.
4. Eruptions of measles, variola, varicella, and scarlatina.

Surgery.

1. Describe fracture of the neck of the femur, giving causes, nature, symptoms, and treatment.
2. Give briefly the pathology of inflammation.
3. Describe senile gangrene.
4. What is the position of the limb in dorsal dislocation of the femur? Give the manipulation needed for its reduction.
5. What is a mulberry calculus? Give the symptoms of stone in the bladder in a child.
6. What are the symptoms of fracture of the base of the skull?

Obstetrics and Gynæcology.

SENIORS, 1885.

1. Define the external, diagonal, and true conjugate diameter of pelvis. How is a measurement of each taken? What is the average length of each in normal pelvis?
2. Describe vascular bodies situated in vulva and entrance of vagina.
3. Describe the different modes of expulsion of head in vertex, face, and pelvic presentations.
4. Management of third stage of labor.
5. Different forms of puerperal hemorrhage during pregnancy.
6. In a case of complete placenta prævia—at term—hemorrhage before dilatation and commenced, give treatment and management of labor and delivery.
7. Commonest causes of dynsmenorrhœa; symptoms and treatment of any one of the forms enumerated.
8. Diagnosis of intra-mural fibroid; symptoms; treatment.

Hygiene.

1. How is the amount of air in soils estimated?
2. How does the proportion of CO_2 in ground-air vary from that in the atmosphere, and why?
3. What relation have forests to temperature, humidity, and water supply?
4. What is the process of sewage purification within the soil?
5. How is the amount of flow through a pipe of given size during a given time estimated?
6. How is mean velocity estimated?
7. What form of pipe presents the least amount of frictional resistance?
8. Describe furnace, steam, and water methods of warming, and the hygienic natures of each.
9. Give usual tests for nitrites and nitrates, and state what the presence of these have in water indicates.
10. What effect has altitude on the respiratory function?
11. What is the combined climatic effect of heat and moisture?
12. Describe the movements of a storm centre and its relation to winds.
13. Name the groups of alimentary substances.
14. What will constitute a perfect diet?

Examination questions, Woman's Medical College of the New York Infirmary (1885). New York Infirmary/Beekman Downtown Hospital

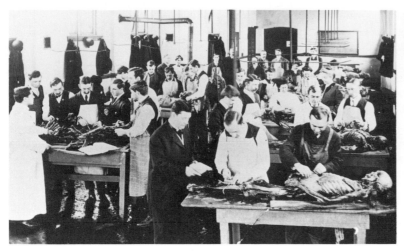

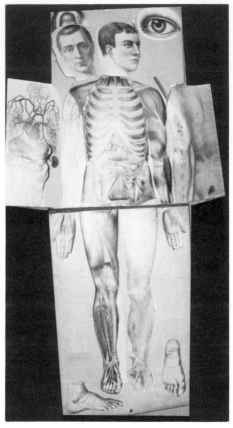

Right: *Dr. Frances Emily White's physiological manikin (c. 1885).* ASCWM, MCP. Above left: *Anatomy lab, Philadelphia College of Osteopathy (c. 1908).* Philadelphia College of Osteopathic Medicine.

to the New York Infirmary Woman's Medical College Class of 1885 were sections on obstetrics and gynecology ("Describe the different modes of expulsion of head in vertex, face, and pelvic presentations"; "In a case of complete placenta praevia—at term—hemorrhage before dilatation has commenced, give treatment and management of labor and delivery"; "Commonest causes of dysmenorrhoea; symptoms and treatment of any one of the forms enumerated"); hygiene ("What is the process of sewage purification within the soil?"; "Give usual tests for nitrites and nitrates, and state what the presence of these in water indicates"; What will constitute a perfect diet?"); and children's Diseases ("Eruption of measles—differentiate it from variola and varicella"; "Anterior polio-myelitis—pathology, degeneration, reaction"; "Relative size of fontanelles at different periods").[3]

While most women physicians taught in "regular" medical schools, some occasionally taught in "irregular" institutions without compromising their careers. In 1904, Class of 1879 graduate Sarah Cohen (May) received a second degree from the Philadelphia College of Osteopathy, where she lectured in anatomy. Other institutions providing more common sources of employment for women physicians included nursing schools. Among the Class of 1879 graduates, Dr. Sophia Presley taught at the New Jersey Training School for Nurses.

The women's medical colleges took as their special responsibility not only the education of women nurses and physicians, but also the public they would eventually serve. As early as 1852, the Woman's Medical College began taking "special students" to study the principles of medicine, hygiene, and women's health, asserting that acquisition of such knowledge was a duty all women "owe to their own offspring [and to] posterity."[4] By 1887, the college's offerings for nonmatriculating students included courses in chemistry, anatomy, physiology, microscopy, and histology. In the fall semester, seven women, mostly married and with children, enrolled in the program.

The women's medical colleges thus served a broad base of functions within the women's medical movement. They educated not only women physicians, but also the doctors who would teach them. They provided the preceptors who would continue training the medical school graduates after they entered private and institutional practice, and they trained the general public in the basics of medical knowledge and preventive care. It was with mixed results, therefore, that the women's medical movement gained its largest goal toward the end of the century—acceptance of women medical students into formerly all-male institutions. For while, in the decade of the 1890s, it seemed women would at last be integrated into mainstream American medical education and clinical training, it was equally clear that the female medical training faculty would not.

As late as 1892, 63 percent of all women enrolled in regular medical schools attended all-female institutions.[5] But as these institutions closed and/or merged with male medical schools, the opportunities for women to hold faculty po-

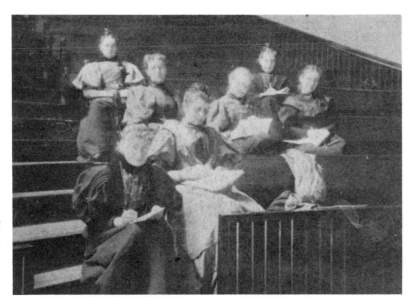

Students in lecture hall, Woman's Medical College of Pennsylvania (c. 1889). ASCWM, MCP.

sitions were sharply curtailed. Dr. Emily Blackwell noted the trend with some concern in her address before the last graduating class of the Woman's Medical College of the New York Infirmary, which its trustees closed in 1899 as Cornell Medical School opened its medical department to women. The closing of the New York Infirmary Woman's Medical School "cut short the teaching careers of a group of capable and rising young women teachers," Blackwell observed.[6] She was prescient as well. Thirteen years later, Cornell did not have a single woman on its teaching staff or in its clinical service.

Coeducation had ironically brought with it the loss of one of the most productive and influential aspects of women physicians' work—medical school teaching—and the attendant loss for female medical students of women faculty as role models and guides.

"Before popular audiences of women . . ."

If opportunities for women physicians to teach in formal settings declined as the century ended, opportunities for women to educate general audiences did not. Throughout the nineteenth century, and into the twentieth, women physicians continued to lecture to and write for ladies' societies, political interest groups, and reform movements. Their motivation combined a Victorian ideology urging them to educate and reform society and their scientific ability as physicians to positively improve conditions affecting life and health. Their topics were those of the women's medical movement: the health of women and children, public health and sanitation, family hygiene, diet and nutrition, and the habits of pure and moral living.

The Woman's Medical College Class of 1879 contributed heavily to the public education effort. Among its twenty graduates, over half are recorded as regularly speaking before women's groups and popular audiences. Dr. Sophia Howard began her lecturing career within six months of her graduation from medical school. Speaking before the Juvenile Temperance Union of Fairport, New York, she

> gave a very interesting address to the children relative to the effects of alchohol upon the stomach and its neighbors. She exhibited specimens and illustrated, by blackboard and crayon, the relative position of the lungs, breast, liver, and stomach, giving the children a clear idea of the circulation of the blood by which means alchoholic poison is conveyed through the system.
>
>   Those present were delighted and profited. Let us hope Miss Howard will spend such an hour often with the children. This organization is exerting a quiet but healthy influence among the youth of our village.[7]

A year later, Harriet Belcher gave an equally positive report of the reception her lectures received. After speaking before a woman's group in Pawtucket, Rhode Island, in 1880, she observed to a friend,

> The audience . . . of all social grades . . . [is] anxious to know all we can tell them about how to take care of their houses, their children, and themselves. I hope [this] may be the starting point of a great deal more. Women can do far

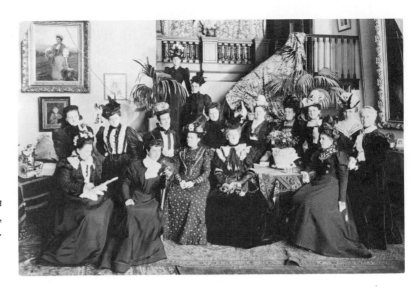

Meeting of Daughters of American Revolution (1898). Bryon collection, Museum of the City of New York.

more then anyone else to help other women. And there are some prominent women here who seem to have that idea.[8]

Throughout the remainder of the century and into the next, the Class of 1879 graduates continued to lecture and to educate. Their topics generally remained within the sphere of the interests of women's medicine. Two years before her death, Eleanor Galt (Simmons) was still arguing her case for family hygiene and preventive medicine in the home:

> Dr. Simmons gave a talk on sanitation in the household. She traced the evolution of our sanitary ideas, and defined the noxious and dangerous elements we have to contend with. Her explanation of personal sanitation, the method of eliminating poisons from the human system, was listened to with intense interest. She emphasized the necessity of burning all materials connected with infectious disease. The club members all felt they had spent a beneficial afternoon. Tea and cake were served.[9]

As nineteenth-century women physicians reached and educated general audiences through their speaking appearances, so they targeted an even wider audience through their publications. In 1897 Dr. Clara Marshall, dean of the Woman's Medical College of Pennsylvania, printed a list of articles published and/or read before medical societies by alumnae of the college.[10] She recorded over five hundred papers, including articles on anaesthesia in surgery, complications in pregnancy, progress in prison reform, care of destitute pregnant women, and an article published by Class of 1879 member Henrietta Louisa Exton on "Some Popular Fallacies in Discussions on Vegetarianism." The article, appearing in the October 1893 issue of *The Hygienic Review* in London, stands typical of the arguments made for a variety of causes by nineteenth-century women physicians. Combining her medical expertise with her direct interest in specific behavioral and health-related reform, Exton wove the scientific, biblical, and moral argument into one. She wrote,

Meat is by no means necessary for a large proportion of the population. Individuals become stronger, lighter and happier as well as better tempered and manifestly healthier upon a diet of cereal foods and vegetable produce, including fruit with a fair condition of eggs and milk and little of other animal food than fish.

[On] the moral side of the question, the flesh eater asserts that certain animals are, on Biblical authority, intended for our sustenance. But let him study the life history of the steak before him [including] its ordeal in the slaughter house, and let him judge whether it conflicts with Scripture's commendation on mercy.[11]

From vegetarianism to sanitation to basic information about disease management and preventive medicine, the information offered by nineteenth-century women physicians helped further their own goals of reforming society and reconstituting the health of its members. If teaching was a work for which women were preeminently fitted, it was also an integral aspect of medicine itself, particularly as defined by nineteenth-century women doctors. Though women physicians did continue to lecture and write for popular audiences well into the twentieth century, the loss of formal medical faculty positions for women professors at the turn of the century cut deeply into the success and future of the women's medical movement. Though women would continue to teach and write and lecture for their reform causes and political goals, the twentieth century would see more of it done through regular school teaching, social work, and nursing. With the decline of women medical professors came a parallel decline in the number of women with medical degrees.[12]

NOTES

1. Rachel Bodley, *Valedictory Address to the Twenty-Ninth Graduating Class of the Woman's Medical College of Pennsylvania,* March 17, 1881 (Philadelphia: 1881), 7.
2. Annual Announcement. Woman's Medical College of Pennsylvania, 1876–1877.
3. Woman's Medical College of the New York Infirmary, "Examination Questions for 1885," 23–25, in Annual Announcement, 1886.
4. Third Annual Announcement, Woman's Medical College of Pennsylvania, 1852.
5. Mary Roth Walsh, *"Doctors Wanted: No Women Need Apply": Sexual Barriers in the Medical Profession, 1835–1975* (New Haven, CT: Yale University Press, 1977), 262.
6. Ibid., 263.
7. Fairport [New York] *Herald Mail,* October 17, 1879.
8. Harriet Belcher to Eliza Johnson, Feb. 9, 1880. Alice McCone Collection.
9. Minutes of the Housekeeper's Club, Coconut Grove, Florida, January 10, 1907. Mrs. Gifford Corres, secretary. Historical Association of Southern Florida.
10. Clara Marshall, *The Woman's Medical College of Pennsylvania: An Historical Outline* (Philadelphia: 1897).
11. H. Louisa Exton. "Some Popular Fallacies in Discussions on Vegetarianism," *The Hygienic Review* (October 1893), 331.
12. See Walsh, *"Doctors Wanted,"* table 6: 193, and discussion.

Institutions

Wide and Fruitful Fields

Ellen J. Smith

The record of the work accomplished by the woman practitioner as Resident or Visiting Physician in Hospital, Asylum, Charitable Institution, College or School for Girls is inspiriting. 60 of 159 are thus engaged. Many mention being physician, usually without salary, to "erring woman's refuge," "orphan's home," or "Reformatory Home for Girls."
–Dr. Rachel Bodley, Dean
Survey of the Living Graduates of the Woman's
Medical College of Pennsylvania, 1881

List of Class of '79 Institutional Affiliations

Avery: Nursery & Child's Hospital, Staten Island, New York
　　　Philadelphia Hospital, Insane Department
　　　Portland Hospital, Portland, Maine
　　　Blockley Hospital, Philadelphia
Baldwin: New England Hospital for Women and Children
　　　　Chicago Hospital for Women
Belcher: New England Hospital
　　　　Pacific Dispensary, California
Cohen: The Sheltering Arms of Philadelphia
Dunn: Ladies of the Maccabees
Flagler: Nursery and Child's Hospital, Staten Island, New York
　　　　General Hospital, Monroe County, Pennsylvania

171

Galt: Nursery and Child's Hospital, Staten Island, New York
Florida School
Lake Placid School
Howard: New England Hospital for Women and Children
Kugler: Founder, Guntur Hospital for Women and Children; Pennsylvania
State Hospital for the Insane, Norristown, Pa., Woman's Hospital,
Philadelphia.
Nicol: New England Hospital
Presley: Woman's Hospital, Philadelphia
Colored Orphan Asylum, Camden, New Jersey
Rhodes: Founder, Highland Home
Richardson: Founder, West Philadelphia Hospital for Women
Schneider: Woman's Hospital, Philadelphia
Wolfenden: New England Hospital
Nursery and Child's Hospital, Staten Island, New York
Wood: Nursery and Child's Hospital, Staten Island, New York

Pennsylvania State Hospital for the Insane

Norristown, Pennsylvania

Throughout the second half of the nineteenth century, the men and women allied with the women's medical movement organized and established institutions providing social and medical care for female patients and children and providing clinical training grounds for the women physicians who would attend to them. Such institutions emerged usually in the form of women's and children's hospitals or specialty centers for pediatric and maternity cases. Rarer were instances of women physicians and women's divisions opening within already established hospital systems. But at the Pennsylvania State Hospital for the Insane, with the creation of a new facility near Norristown, an unusual instance of an older institution integrating the concerns and directions of a female medical department occurred.

The hospital opened its doors on July 12, 1880, the newest of five facilities in the Pennsylvania mental hospital system. From its inception, Norristown was an innovative institution. Situated in Pennsylvania's rolling hill country, the physical plant employed an experimental "separate building plan . . . entirely new and untried until now." Seven buildings housed separate departments, residences, and treatment areas, "conducted as though they were independent hospitals . . . provided for from a common kitchen."[1] The attendant advantages of more privacy, light, air, and ventilation within the individual buildings and resulting improvements in patient health and cleanliness immediately impressed the staff and trustees. Within its second full year of operation, the facility expanded further, acquiring additional paved roads, a sewer system, landscape grading for drainage, an eight-foot fence, a barn, and a root house that doubled as a gate house.

The independent building plan led to a second conscious innovation at the site. With the Women's Department now housed in its own plant, an entirely female medical and supervisory staff was employed to treat the female pa-

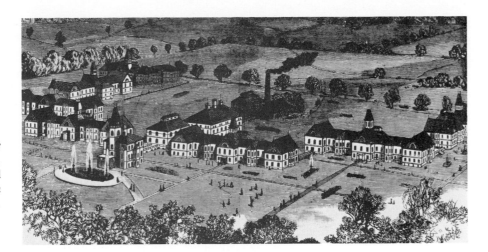

Sketch of Norristown State Hospital by S. F. Yeager, Frank Leslie's Illustrated Newspaper, *Lutheran Church of America. August 14, 1880.*

tients, removing any possibility of abuse or immodest behavior in treating the women by male patients or staff. With the strong urging of Dr. Hiram Corson, Quaker physician and long-time supporter of the women's medical movement, Dr. Alice Bennett, a graduate of the Woman's Medical College of Pennsylvania was appointed head of the Women's Department, the first woman in the nation to direct a female division in a mental institution. The nineteenth-century argument that women physicians were most appropriate and able to treat women patients was acknowledged for the first time at the level of a major state medical institution.

In late 1880, Dr. Bennett was joined on the Norristown staff by Woman's Medical College Class of 1879 graduate Dr. Anna Kugler. Appointed as first assistant physician in the Women's Department, Kugler served with Bennett for just over two years before accepting a permanent missionary post in India. The 1882 Annual Report for the State Hospital for the Insane at Norristown gives a good sense of the character of medicine and mental health management Bennett and Kugler practiced at Norristown within the sturcture of the state mental health system.

Though a new facility, Norristown was already overcrowded by its second full year of operation. An 1881 census of 748 patients had swollen to 950 patients housed in seven buildings by the end of 1882.[2] The Women's Department alone showed an increase in resident population from 367 in September 1881 to 457 in September 1882.[3] "This increase," wrote Dr. Bennett,

has necessarily crowded our wards far beyond their estimated capacity, beyond what had been supposed compatible with health and safety, and has been the source of an amount of care and anxiety for those in charge not to be estimated. Under these circumstances it is peculiarly gratifying again to report a year of general good health and prosperity, free from serious accident or suicide, and free from all contagious or infectious disease, with a percentage of deaths slightly lower, and of recoveries higher, than in the preceeding year.[4]

Bennett had cause to be grateful. As a state institution, Norristown received a high percentage of charity cases, cases private physicians and institutions could no longer handle, and a disproportionately low subsidy from the state underwriting the patient population.[5] In addition to treating the mental health of her patients, she and Dr. Kugler were responsible for the physical health of the residents, attending to their medical and surgical needs as well. With one attendant for every twelve patients, Bennett and Kugler managed a large department, already overcrowded, understaffed, and underfunded. That they had avoided acute, contagious, and infectious outbreaks, Bennett "considered a tribute to good sanitary conditions" and "somewhat remarkable."[6]

Still, the patient population at Norristown continued to increase. Admission was fairly simple, requiring only certification of the patient's condition by two or more reputable physicians and a "Form of Application" filled out and signed by the patient's legal guardian, a relative, or a friend. Application questions drew information about the patient's general health, her family status, her family's medical and mental health history, and a detailed account of the patient's current symptoms, personal habits, and treatment she may have received to date for the illness.[7] Of the 212 admissions for 1881–82, the "Apparent Causes of Insanity" for 115 of them were recorded as "Physical Causes," including "puerperal [fever] (22 cases); intemperance and other excesses (16 cases); epilepsy (12 cases); debility from overwork (12 cases);

FORM OF APPLICATION.

The friends of patients making application for admission into the State Hospital for the Insane of the South-eastern District of Pennsylvania, are requested, with the assistance of the family physician, to annex full and complete answers to the following questions:—

1. What is the patient's name?
   What is the age?
   Is . . . single or married?
2. Where was . . . born?
   Where is . . . present residence?
3. What is . . . occupation?
   If a female, that of the husband or father?
4. When did the first symptoms of insanity occur, and in what manner?
5. Is this the first attack? If others, when, and what were their duration?
6. Has the patient any permanent hallucination? and what is its nature?
7. Has the patient any disposition to injure others? If so, is it from premeditation or sudden passion?
8. Does the propensity to suicide exist? Has the patient ever made an attempt? If so, in what manner?
9. Has the patient a disposition to destroy clothing, furniture, &c.? Is the patient cleanly in . . . habits?
10. What was the patient's natural disposition? Was there any peculiarity or eccentricity?
11. Have any members of the family ever been insane? On the father's or mother's side?
12. Has the patient ever been addicted to the intemperate use of intoxicating drinks, opium or tobacco? Does the patient indulge in any improper habits?
13. Has the patient ever had an injury of the head, epilepsy, or any hereditary disease, sudden suppression of any eruption or accustomed discharge?

14. What is the cause of the attack?
15. Has any restraint or confinement been resorted to? If so, of what kind, and for how long?
16. Has the patient received any medical treatment? Has . . . been bled, cupped or blistered?
17. State any other particulars of the patient's history which may have a bearing on the present attack.

☞ "That insane persons may be placed in a Hospital for the Insane by their legal guardians, or by their relatives or friends, in case they have no guardians, but never without the certificate of two or more reputable physicians, after a personal examination, made within one week of the date thereof, and this certificate to be duly acknowledged and sworn to or affirmed before some magistrate or judicial officer, who shall certify to the genuineness of the signatures, and to the respectability of the signers."—*Law of April, 1869.*

FORM OF PHYSICIAN'S CERTIFICATE.

WE. . . . . of . . . . in the county of . . . . do certify that we have this day seen and personally examined . . . . of . . . . in the county of . . . . and believe . . . . . . to be insane and a proper patient to be sent to the Trustees of the State Hospital for the Insane of the South-eastern District of Pennsylvania.

. . . . *M. D.*
. . . . *M. D.*
. . . . 188 . .

I, ... of . . . . in the county of . . . . do certify that the above certificate has been sworn to, or affirmed, before me, and that the signatures are genuine and the signers are respectable physicians of . . . .

. . . . [L. S.]
. . . . 188 . .

Form of Application, Annual Report, State Hospital for the Insane, Norristown, Pennsylvania, 1881–82. NYAM. Page 2 of Form of Application.

TABLE XII.—*Number of the Attack of those Admitted.*

	For the Year.	From the Beginning.
1st Attack	165	492
2d "	12	39
3d "	2	11
4th "	2	3
5th "	1	2
6th "	2	2
Unknown	28	132
Total	212	681

TABLE XIII.—*Apparent Causes of Insanity.*

	For the Year.	From the Beginning.
PHYSICAL CAUSES.		
Acute Febrile Disease	6	13
Apoplexy	4	9
Brain Tumors	1	1
Burn	1	1
Congenital	9	19
Change of Climate		2
Debil'y from Chronic Disease	11	35
" " Over-work	12	20
" " Lactation	2	3
Epilepsy	12	28
Exhaustion of Travel	1	1
Heat-stroke		4
Injury to Head	2	7
Intemp. and other excesses	16	30
Malaria	3	3
Marriage		1
Menopause	3	8
Puberty	2	8
Puerperal	22	43
Senility	5	18
Suppressio Mensuim		2
Uterine Disease	3	4
Total Physical Causes	115	263
MORAL CAUSES.		
Anxiety		5
Domestic Unhappiness	2	23
Disappointment	2	5

TABLE XIII.—CONTINUED.

Financial Trouble	2	7
Grief	7	22
Homesickness		2
Jealousy		2
Loss of Property		1
Loss of Occupation		1
Loss of Sight		1
Mental Stroke		4
Religious Excitement	2	8
Solitary Life	1	1
Spiritualism	1	1
Trouble	5	26
Total Moral Causes	22	109
Total Physical Causes	115	263
No Manifest Cause	45	45
Unknown	30	264
Total	212	681

TABLE XIV.—*Duration of Disease before Admission.*

	For the Year.	From the Beginning.
Congential	9	19
Under 3 months	45	101
3 to 6 months	13	49
6 to 12 months	20	54
1 to 2 years	16	79
2 to 3 years	18	61
3 to 4 years	14	53
4 to 5 years	5	23
5 to 10 years	24	102
10 to 15 years	10	35
15 to 20 years	5	18
20 to 30 years	8	24
30 years and over	2	5
Unknown	23	58
Total	212	681

TABLE XV.—*Heredity.*

	For the Year.	From the Beginning.
Insanity in Family	70	191
No Insanity in Family	88	253
History not known	54	237
Total	212	681

Left: *Apparent Causes of Insanity, Annual Report, State Hospital for the Insane, Norristown, Pennsylvania.* NYAM. Right above: *Page 2 of Apparent Causes.*

and debility from chronic disease (11 cases.)" Twenty-two patients were admitted for "Moral Causes," including grief (7 cases); trouble (5 cases); and religious excitement, domestic unhappiness, disappointment, and financial trouble (2 cases each.)[8] But cautioning against too much clinical reliance on attributed "causes of insanity," Dr. Bennett noted that an admitting diagnosis was less an indicator of patient prognosis than the "quality" of the brain (mind) the patient possessed.

> A table of "Causes of Insanity" must always be unsatisfactory and unsafe as a basis of reasoning. Even assuming that it is made up from histories given without error or reservation, it does not take into account the *quality* of brain with which we have to deal, and which is as varied and uncertain as the influences operating upon it.
>
> The same circumstance which is a veritable "cause of insanity" in a brain weak by inheritance or by indulgence, may be only an incident to another more fortunate or better trained.[9]

The majority of women admitted to Bennett's and Kugler's care were between twenty and forty years old and seemed to be primarily working-class women: wives of laborers and mechanics, or women who were themselves domestics or in the needle trades.[10] Admitting diagnoses included mania (acute and chronic), 50 percent; melancholia (acute and chronic) 15 percent; dementia (acute, chronic, and senile) 23 percent; epilepsy 8 percent; imbecility and idiocy 6 percent; and paresis 1 percent.[11] Patient histories divided about evenly between those with known cases of insanity in the family, those without such family histories, and those where family histories were unknown.[12]

More important to patient prognosis than admitting diagnosis or heredity, from Dr. Bennett's point of view, was the length of time a patient had been ill before she was admitted. Approximately 21 percent of patients admitted to the Norristown Women's Department arrived within three months of the onset of their illness. Another 15 percent arrived within the first year. Twenty-three percent came within one to four years of onset, and another 16 percent arrived five to fifteen years into the disease.[13] Chances for improvement or cure were directly related to the length of time a patient had been ill before she came to Norristown.

> The importance of *early* hospital treatment cannot be too often repeated and emphasized. . . . So often friends come to us and say: "We have kept her at home *as long as we could;* and so often we have seen such patients for whom treatment has been delayed for some months, fail to recover when . . . they should have done so. . . . *Change* is the most important element of treatment.[14]

Among the 573 patients under her care at some point in 1881–82, 44 cases of recovery and discharge were recorded by Dr. Bennett. All who recovered were patients at Norristown less than two years, and nearly half had been there less than six months.[15] Another 13 patients were discharged "much improved," and 19 were discharged "improved" (of whom 3 were subsequently readmitted).[16] Thirty-six patients died during the year from a variety of physical as well as mental ailments.[17] Overall, 86 patients under Bennett's and Kugler's care left Norristown improved, or about 1 in every 7 patients.

In the treatment of her charges, Alice Bennett seems to have employed a reform-minded style of managing mental health patients. She was particularly adamant against use of behavior-altering drugs and physical restraints. In 1882, an average of only nine patients per day received doses of "hypnotics."[18] On the subject of physical restraints, Bennett gave no quarter at all:

> I am led to believe that much of the paraphernalia of the approved Hospital for the Insane—heavily barred windows, massive, immovable furniture and the like—has too much the tendency to surround the patient with an atmosphere of suspicion, against which he naturally places himself. . . .[19]

> No mechanical restraint has been made use of during the year. . . . *I believe the use of mechanical restraint to be absolutely incompatible with any influence for good.* . . . [Its use] is always a confession of *failure.*[20]

Bennett opted rather for treatment that encouraged independence and self-esteem and which, through its humane example, would elicit behaviors of kindness and civility in the patients:

> While those having homicidal or suicidal tendencies are protected with the utmost

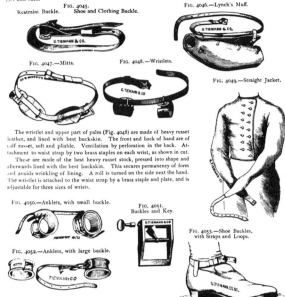

Restraints for the Insane. Illustration from the 1889 George Tiemann medical instrument catalogue. Lane Medical Library, Stanford University Medical Center.

vigilance, the great mass of patients are allowed much liberty, the tranquilizing effects of which are constantly being seen.[21]

MEDICAL.		SURGICAL.		GYNÆCOLOGICAL.	
Ague	3	Abscess	6	No. patients examined for Uterine or Ovarian Disease	100
Arthritis	1	Anthrax	1	No. treated for same	42
Bronchitis	25	Dislocation (Lower Maxilla)	1	No. benefited by treatment	38
Bright's Disease	6	Fissue of Anus	1	No. now under regular treatment	22
Conjunctivitis	10	Fracture of Radius	1	Lacerations of Cervix	14
Diarrhoea	35	Fed with Nasal Tube, (No. of *persons*)	36	" of Perineum	24
Dysentery	5	Fed with Œsophageal Tube	1	" of Cervix and Perin.	25
Dysuria	2	Sprain of Wrist	1	Prolapsus Uteri	6
Enteritis, Chronic	2	Sprain of Ankle	1	Lateral Displacements	7
Eczema	4	Teeth Extracted	53	Anterior "	9
Erysipelas	3	Vaccinations	440	Posterior "	13
Gastric Ulcer	1	Venesections	7	Hypertrophy of Uterus	3
Hemorrhoids	7			Chronic Cellulitis	10
Heart Disease	3			Endocervicitis	14
Intermittent Fever	13			Vaginitis	5
Indigestion	43			Operation for Procidentia Ut., (Le Fort)	1
Keratitis	1			Operation for Lacerations of Perin.	1
Neuralgia	5				
Otitis	2				
Pharyngitis	5				
Pneumonia, Acute	2	Average daily No. Patients taking Hypnotics for last 8 Months of the Year.			
Pleurisy, Acute	1	No. Patients taking Chloral Hydrate			2.15
Phthisis	15	" " " Bromide of Potassium			1.18
Pyæmia	1	" " " Hyoscyamine			4.98
Rheumatism	3	" " " Morphine			1.30
Rhus Poisoning	4	" " " Conium			.07
Sciatica	1				
Stomatitis	1	Total			9.00
Tonsillitis	1				
Urticaria	1				

Record of General Medical and Surgical Work, Annual Report, State Hospital for the Insane, Norristown, Pennsylvania, 1881–82. NYAM.

INSTITUTIONS

One who has watched the transformation of cases like these under the influence of personal liberty and rational methods of treatment, can but marvel that a principle so plain—so evidently founded in the commonest laws of our common nature—should admit of discussion.[22]

And so Norristown patients were encouraged to make visits home, to engage in "productive" occupations like housework, sewing, and knitting while at the hospital, and to take advantage of the fresh air and the beautiful grounds. Bennett made special note of the holiday celebrations the Women's Department sponsored to draw the patients together.[23] As the first female to direct a Women's Department in a state mental institution, Alice Bennett profited from the Victorian notion that as a woman physician, she could best treat patients of her own sex. Bennett, in her turn, introduced her own ideas of patient management: mental and physical care mixed with a nurturing atmosphere that recreated a "proper" home environment as closely as possible. Her idea of simultaneously nurturing and reforming and healing was born of the women's medical movement and welcomed in the reform-minded and experimental setting of the Norristown State Hospital for the Insane.

Nursery and Child's Hospital, Country Branch

Staten Island, New York

The nineteenth-century women's medical movement consciously chose as its mission the improvement of medical care available to women, expectant mothers, and children. Among its particular focuses were the worthy poor of the populous lower classes, people who had little access to hospitals, physicians, or regular medical treatment. As graduates of the women's medical colleges researched and improved treatment in obstetrics, gynecology, and pediatrics, they joined other women and men in establishing permanent institutions that not only specialized in these branches of medicine, but also created entire environments where the interlocking goals of social, religious, and medical reform of their clientele could be accomplished. Almost entirely creations of the second half of the nineteenth century, these institutions not only cured and cared for a previously neglected patient population, but also provided clinical and postgraduate training experience for physicians allied to the women's medical programs. Among the earliest of the institutions founded to care exclusively for women and children was the Nursery and Child's Hospital of New York, established after a series of newspaper articles exposed the horrors of baby farming and the ill treatment of infants at the city's almshouses.

The Nursery and Child's Hospital was founded in 1854 to provide for infants of wet nurses who were being left improperly cared for while their own mothers nursed the children of well-to-do women. Originally located in a large Federal-style house on Sixth Avenue at Fifteenth Street in New York City, the facility soon expanded its purposes to include care for a broad range of sick children and expectant mothers. When the hospital relocated to larger quarters on Lexington Avenue at Fifty-first Street, it encompassed a children's hospital, a maternity center, and a foster care and adoption agency.

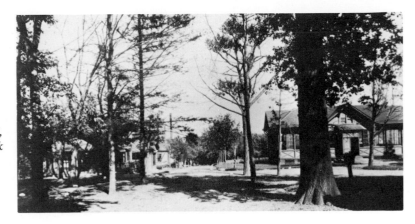

Grounds of the Nursery and Child's Hospital, Country Branch, Staten Island, New York (c. 1890). Cornell Medical Center.

In 1870, the Nursery and Child's Hospital opened a Country Branch on Staten Island, and it was in that location that at least five 1879 graduates of the Woman's Medical College—Mary Alice Avery, Phoebe Flagler, Eleanor Galt, Mary Wolfenden, and Mina Fitch Wood—served on the nursery and child's staff. The branch was an innovative facility, consisting of a main hospital and a series of fresh-air children's villages where children lived in groups in cottages, attended by resident matrons. The Country Branch provided adult supervision, schools, religious guidance, food, clothing, and medical care to the children it admitted. The facility was largely self-sufficient, taking its water from a clear spring on the property and raising a fair proportion of the produce consumed by the patients and staff. The institution kept dairy cows, pigs, and chickens to provide milk, meat, and eggs year-round and supplemented its stores with purchases and donations from supporters of the institution.

Admission to the Country Branch was generally limited to infants and children under four years of age. Expectant or newly delivered mothers were required to nurse at least one orphaned baby in addition to their own. (Women whose children died were required to nurse two infants.) Children admitted had to be free of contagious disease, vaccinated, and provided with shoes and a dozen diapers (where applicable) by their parents or guardians. The fee for infants was ten dollars per month; children who could walk were charged seven dollars; and hospital or sick children were charged nine dollars per month. Parents were allowed to visit their children "once in a fortnight, between 10 A.M. and 3 P.M."[24]

By 1880, the year the Class of 1879 graduates began staffing the Country Branch, the hospital had grown into a large and well-managed institution. Except for associated visiting physicians and male laborers on the premises, the facility was entirely staffed and managed by women. A massive repair and building program had just been completed, including painting and refurbishing the main hospital and most of the cottages and a massive plumbing installation that brought water and gas to the sanitarium. In keeping with the social as well as medical aims of the institution, a "small room where the men in our employ" could retire at the end of the day was opened. "By providing books and papers," the directress wrote, "we hope to prevent all desire to frequent places where liquor can be obtained."[25]

In the fresh air of rural New York City, expectations ran high that medical

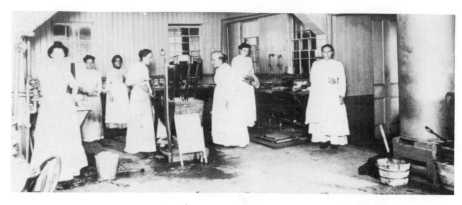

Laundry room, Nursery and Child's Hospital, Country Branch, Staten Island, New York (c. 1890). Cornell Medical Center.

improvement would accrue to the Nursery and Child's residents. Census figures generally matched such optimism. The Medical Report for the year ending March 1, 1880, indicated "no epidemics of scarlet fever or measles—and all the wards in the Institution are at present in excellent condition."[26]

> During the year 149 children, 201 pregnant women, and 38 [wet] nurses were admitted, and 155 infants born. The total number of children [treated] in the institution was 520; of which 205 remain, 62 died, 3 were stillborn, and 246 were discharged, accordingly the death rate was 11.9 per cent. The death rate [the preceeding year was] 10.55 per cent.[27]

Most of the children who died at the Country Branch were under one year old; only two children over the age of two succumbed during the year covered by the report. But two years later, the institution was not so lucky.

> Diphtheria swept through the hospital in the spring. We performed three trachiatomies, one of them satisfactorily. They stopped using the well water because it was infected. After one child died of small pox, we re-vaccinated the entire hospital population. We had to close down the lying in ward for two months when we could not stop a rash of puerperal fever.[28]

In general, however, the Country Branch hospital boasted an overall excellent recovery record. The institution also prided itself on finding fitting placement for its abandoned or orphaned children. In 1880 the resident physician reported

> . . . we have sent seven [children] to the west by the Children's Aid Society. Eight have gone to the House of Industry, in Worth Street, to learn trades. One has entered the home for Ruptured and Crippled. One was received at St. Johnland. Three of the blind children who came to us from the Alms House have entered the Blind Asylum. Three have been adopted. The rest of those discharged returned to parents or guardians.[29]

Unplaced children in the institution reaching five years of age were automatically assigned to "village homes and . . . school[s]." There, it was assumed, the children would grow up in a normal home environment "with self-respect and no feelings of pauperism."[30] Social as well as physical resti-

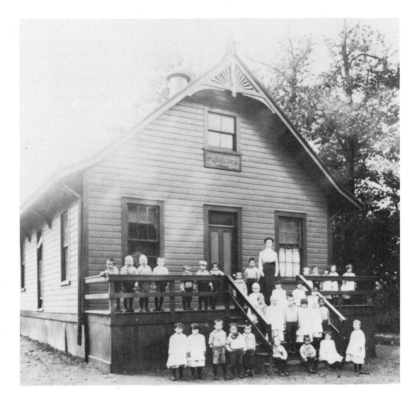

Orphans with matron on steps of cottage Nursery and Child's Hospital, Country Branch, Staten Island, New York (c. 1890). Medical Archives, New York Hospital, Cornell Medical Center.

tution was part of the program of regular care at the Nursery and Child's Hospital, as it was throughout the institutions allied with the nineteenth-century women's medical movement.

The Nursery and Child's Hospital worked hard in other ways as well to turn its residents into respectable women. With 64 percent of all births taking

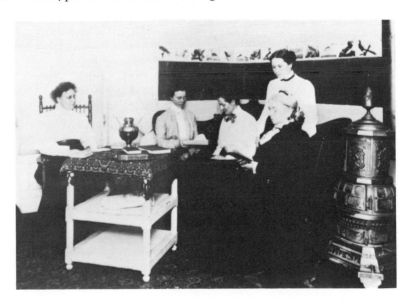

Medical staff meeting at Nursery and Child's Hospital, Country Branch, Staten Island, New York. Cornell Medical Center.

place being illegitimate,[31] the Hospital was adamant that women giving birth out-of-wedlock for the second or subsequent times could not be admitted to the institution:

> We receive mothers, deserted by their husbands, and women who have hitherto lived virtuous lives, but come for shelter, when suffering remorse for sin. Our rules forbid our taking women who bring a second illegitimate child into the world. And this rule must be rigidly enforced. It requires constant vigilance, that no evil association can contaminate those whom we hope to restore to a virtuous life.[32]

The simultaneous goals of restoring women and children to physical health while influencing them toward moral well-being characterized the nineteenth-century women's medical movement and the institutions created by it. Guided by ideology that assured women of their naturally sympathetic and healing natures, Nursery and Child's directress Mary A. DuBois argued within the stream of the women's medical and reform movements when she wrote, in "cases of women and children in general . . . it seems their care should be given to women":

> We should recollect that as women have to bear *all* the suffering, opprobrium and scorn, they should be shielded by those who feel the injustice which condemns women alone. Female physicians are obliged to pass as strict examinations as men, before they graduate. With the learning and skill which so many have already exhibited, it is time that an earnest plea should be made that our *Public City Institutions* for women and children, should be placed under the care and guidance of Women Physicians.[33]

The Nursery and Child's Hospital, following its own recommendations, did just that, providing, in its country setting, training for two generations of women physicians and facilities for mothers and children to regain their health, their self-respect, and each other.

Chicago Hospital for Women and Children

Chicago, Illinois

Throughout most of the second half of the nineteenth century, women physicians found few professional appointments or privileges open to them in existing medical clinics, dispensaries, hospitals, and institutions. As in the creation of separate women's medical schools, male and female supporters of the women's medical movement began, after the Civil War, to establish institutions in which women doctors could practice, train new doctors and nurses, and create an environment they felt appropriate to treating the people who made up the bulk of their patient population: women and children. Between 1857 and 1895 hospitals for women and children were founded throughout the United States, a direct outgrowth of the aims of the women's medical movement. Among the earliest, the best-known, and most successful of these institutions was the Chicago Hospital for Women and Children, founded by Dr. Mary Harris Thompson in February 1865.

Mary Thompson was born in Fort Ann, New York, in 1829 and received her preparatory medical training at the West Poultney Academy in Vermont. After a year of clinical work at the New York Infirmary for Women and Children, she took her medical degree and moved west to Chicago. There, Rush Medical School refused to admit her for advanced training, but Northwestern University Medical School took her (along with three other women) for one year before barring women from attendance for the next fifty years. Thompson, however, was allowed to retain some privileges and to use the school's facilities.[34]

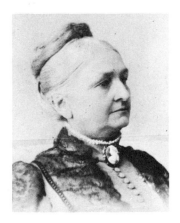

Dr. Mary Harris Thompson, 1829–95, founder of Chicago Hospital for Women and Children. Mary Thompson Hospital.

A tangential affiliation to a medical school, however, could not suffice. The Chicago Mary Thompson found was a city teeming with Civil War refugees, impoverished immigrants from the east, and women and children with little means of care or support. Chicago's two hospitals at the time, Mercy and Marine, were both filled to capacity and did not accept women patients under any circumstances. Neither did they permit women physicians to admit or attend patients in their facilities.

Mary Thompson remedied all of that. On May 8, 1865, the hospital she had organized three months prior—the Chicago Hospital for Women and Children—opened its doors in a large frame house on the corner of Rush and Indiana Streets. The facility specialized in treating the diseases of women and children and consisted of fourteen beds, two rooms for a dispensary, and a small storage room for medicine. Its aims were medical, reformist, and educational, in keeping with the ideology of the women's medical movement:

1st. To afford a home for women and children among the respectable poor in need of medical and surgical treatment.
2nd. To give them such treatment at their homes by an assistant physician.
3rd. To sustain a free dispensary for the benefit of the same class.
4th. To train competent nurses among this class of our population.[35]

The hospital was immediately successful. In its first year 212 patients were admitted, 544 were treated in the dispensary, and 10 patients were treated at their homes. By the end of the year, the hospital had outgrown its quarters

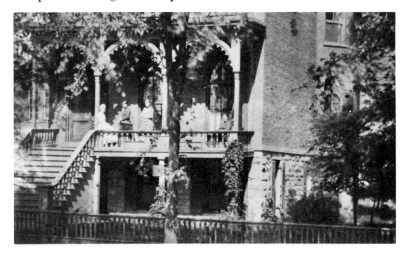

Chicago Hospital for Women and Children, 1871–73, at 598 West Adams, was set up within twenty-four hours after the Great Chicago Fire to treat the wounded. Mary Thompson Hospital.

and moved to 212 Ohio Street, where it remained for the next three years. In 1870, with three thousand dollars and a public campaign to raise ten thousand more, the hospital moved to 402 North State Street, where Thompson believed the institution had found a permanent home. The Great Chicago Fire of 1871 radically altered those plans. The building burned to the ground within five minutes, amazingly injuring no one.

Within twenty-four hours, the Chicago Relief and Aid Society contacted Dr. Thompson and agreed to guarantee maintenance of the hospital if she would immediately reopen it. She did, in a rented house on West Adams Street, "carpeted wtih mattresses and patients from attic to basement. Here helpless women and children—suffering from general sickness, induced by fright, exposure to excessive fatigue, and fire, followed by cold rains—were given food and medicine."[36] Two additional moves brought the hospital to the corner of Paulina and Adams streets by February 1873, purchased with a twenty-five thousand dollar grant from the Relief and Aid Society on the condition that the hospital would care for twenty-five patients a year free of charge. There it was located in 1880 when Class of 1879 graduate Emma Baldwin came to serve.

By the time Dr. Baldwin arrived, Mary Thompson had established one of the leading medical facilities in the country. The 1884 annual report announced the hospital free of debt and with a larger surplus for annual expenses than the year prior.[37] The medical and administrative staff was almost entirely female and enjoyed the cooperation of "the best medical men in the city."[38] The hospital's own staff consisted of medical and surgical physicians, house physicians, a dozen consulting physicians, and a dispensary staff on which Dr. Emma Baldwin served. In the year ending March 1, 1884, the last year Dr. Baldwin seems to have served in the hospital, the staff treated 102 obstetrical cases, delivered 92 infants, treated 93 gynecological cases, performed 41 gynecological surgeries and 12 general surgeries, treated 20 cases in the medical ward, and saw 1,465 patients in the dispensary.[39]

Admission to the hospital was open to "women for confinement, and women and children with any disease not *incurable* or *contagious*."

Admission standards to the hospital indicate its aims to aid those perceived as the deserving poor:

> Respectable women, once living in comfort and ease, but reduced to poverty and sickness have here found a home until restored to health. Good women having homes of their own, have come to the Hospital when almost to become mothers, for the sake of availing themselves of the medical advice and nursing; others at this time have found a refuge here when deserted by husbands who either did not care for them, or were obliged to leave them to seek work.
>   Servant girls without homes, when sick and obliged to give up their situations, have here found shelter, medical care, and good nursing. Sick children, whose parents could bestow little time or attention upon them—being obliged to earn their daily bread—have received at the Hospital the kindest care.[40]

Outpatients found assistance as well. The dispensary, open daily from 7:30 A.M. to 3:00 P.M. provided advice, surgical treatment, and medicines "at a very low price."[41] Patient demands on the dispensary increased each year

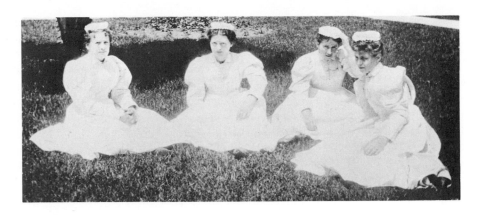

Nellie Wood, Caroline Miller, Irena Orrell, and Ms. Kilgor were 1896 and 1897 graduates of the first training school for nurses in the Midwest, founded by Dr. Mary Harris Thompson in 1874. Mary Thompson Hospital.

Emma Baldwin worked there, with annual visits rising from 389 patients in 1880 to 616 patients by 1884.[42] Though difficult work, dispensary affiliations provided young doctors with broad clinical experience and responsibility and were widely sought-after posts.

Thompson's vision for the hospital also expanded beyond its treatment capacities. In 1870, with Dr. William H. Ryford, she founded and staffed the allied Women's Medical College of Chicago, for the purpose of training women physicians and surgeons. It was the first medical college of women in the Midwest.[43] Four years later, in 1874, Thompson founded the hospital's School for Nurses, the first such facility in Chicago.

Emma Baldwin's last year at the hospital in 1884 was also the last year of the institution at the Adams Street site. The following year, in December 1885, the Chicago Hospital for Women and Children moved to a new five-story brick building with an eighty-patient capacity and quarters for twenty-two nursing students. There the hospital celebrated its thirtieth anniversary on May 8, 1895, with a reception on the hospital grounds. Ten days later Dr. Thompson was still immersed in her usual routine at the hospital. She made rounds, performed two operations, and that evening went to visit friends. The following morning she awoke with a severe headache. She was unconscious by midnight and died two days later of cerebral hemorrhage. Her death was mourned in Chicago, where over a thousand people attended her funeral, and across the nation, where news of her work and achievements had spread. Soon after her death, the Board of Trustees changed the name of the Chicago Hospital for Women and Children to the Mary Thompson Hospital, a name that it bears to this day.[44]

The Sheltering Arms

Philadelphia, Pennsylvania

In 1881, in a German-Jewish immigrant neighborhood in Philadelphia, the Protestant Episcopal Church opened a home at 717 Franklin Street "to care for outcast children, and through them to help their mothers to a better life, honorable in the sight of God and the world."[45] With enormous faith in the morally transforming powers of motherhood, the institution sought to save "the lives of scores of helpless babes," while restoring to their mothers "the holy principle of motherhood, which bewildering passion had almost plucked out of the woman's heart."[46] The best medical care the institution could provide and the gentle influences of good Christian women were to combine to improve the prospects of foundlings, abandoned and neglected children, and the women who either bore them out-of-wedlock or were abandoned by their husbands.

The home setting of the institution was intentional. In an environment where nineteenth-century women were assumed to thrive and set a moral example for their families, the institution's founders hoped to influence mothers fallen away from their innate maternal responsibilities and calling. The home was "to foster maternal love by seeking out the mothers of deserted children, and bring them together in a comfortable home under healthful influences."[47] The house on Franklin Street would "receive the little outcast and aim to preserve a human life of possible future usefulness."[48] With nineteenth-century imagery and accuracy, they called their institution "The Sheltering Arms."

The Sheltering Arms did indeed save the lives of scores of "helpless babes." Foundlings were brought to the home from throughout the area, often by the police. Other infants were left on the steps of the house, or sent from other charities. Still others were discovered by passersby, often, the staff reported, in the better areas of the city. The first annual report noted sadly "that many of the infants were brought to the Institution in actually a dying condition." Some were brought in the last stages of "horrible diseases which could only terminate in early death." Other infants and children were victims of abuse "almost incredible in cruelty." The report went on to conclude that "nearly all the infants received were emaciated by neglect, or constitutionally wrecked by criminal resort to drugs by their unhappy mothers."[49] In the Sheltering Arms, such infants were given one more chance at life.

The people who gave them that chance were men and women active in church work and in the women's medical movement. The Sheltering Arms was one of a number of charities sponsored by the Protestant Episcopal Church in Philadelphia and supported by the staff and graduates of the Woman's Medical College of Pennsylvania. The home's three-tiered system of management included a board of council, gentlemen in charge of finances and internal arrangements of the house; a board of managers, women who had responsibility for the entire management of the home's internal affairs; and a medical board, consisting of four visiting physicians and surgeons with oversight of the facility's sanitation and hygiene programs. In addition, two or three full-time matrons, wet nurses, and an attending physician provided in-house staff to counsel, cure, and console the women and children they took in.

The institution almost immediately realized its founders' aims. In its first eleven months of operation, the home admitted 110 infants. Forty-seven of them were restored to their mothers, 8 were adopted, and 26 remained in the home at the end of the year. Thirty-seven of the infants had died, a relatively low statistic given the condition in which most of the children arrived.[50] The period from November 1, 1883 to January 1, 1885, saw 160 infants treated at the home, plus 94 adults. Of the 54 patients who died, only 8 deaths were attributed to "acute intercurrent disease," while the remaining 46 deaths were linked to "hereditary and incurable diseases."[51] Overall, the home reported a 34 percent mortality rate among its patient population.

But there were periods when the mortality rates were much higher. The summer of 1883 was such a time. In late June, throughout July, and into August, measles swept the infants' wards under a scorching summer heat. Matron S. C. Pearce, who had herself only arrived at the beginning of June, recorded the early signs of the epidemic with grim despair in her diary:[52]

> June 23, 1883: Little Harry Friel died about four o'clock p.m. Alice Fletcher is very sick. I think it is better to send for a wet nurse for her.
> June 24: Annie died 4 o'clock a.m. I will read the burial service over it.
> June 25: Henry Brown died 9 o'clock tonight. Gradual debility or marasmus.
> June 27: Girard Clark died this morning about ½ past 5 o'clock of marasmus. He has been lingering for some time. Willie Kennedy is sick, throwing up. Maybe getting the measles—don't know.
> June 28: Some of the children are complaining. Expect they will take the measles.

The mysterious illnesses and deaths continued, and on June 29, Matron Pearce's worst fears were confirmed as measles were diagnosed. By the first week of July, the epidemic was so extensive that the home's third story was converted into an infirmary:

> July [?]: May Dagar, Kate Roenheld, Frank Langely, Willie Kennedy, Robert McCasidy are all taken with the measles. We now have about ten children down with the measles.

Report of the attending physician, the Sheltering Arms, Philadelphia, January 1885. Historical Society of Pennsylvania.

Report of the Attending Physician.

To the President and Board of Managers of "The Sheltering Arms."

I have the pleasure to submit my Annual Report of the Sheltering Arms, from November 1st, 1883, to January 1st, 1885.

ADMISSIONS.

1883.	ADULTS.	MALE INFANTS.	FEM. INFANTS.	TOTAL
November,	8	8	5	21
December,	2	5	2	9
1884.				
January,	6	1	4	11
February,	3	4	2	9
March,	5	8	6	19
April,	5	6	2	13
May,	6	8	7	21
June,	6	7	4	17
July,	8	9	7	24
August,	13	6	12	31
September,	6	4	9	19
October,	9	5	9	23
November,	9	6	4	19
December,	8	5	5	18
	94	82	78	254

Total number of patients treated during the year, 205, of which 65 were adults, and 140 infants. Total number of deaths, 54. Of these 46 were due to "hereditary" and incurable diseases, while only 8 were due to acute, intercurrent disease.

CAUSES OF DEATH.

Marasmus,	32
Hydrocephalus,	4
Hereditary Syphilis,	6
Inanition,	3
Tubercular Enteritis,	1
Meningitis,	1
Pneumonia,	2
Entero-colitis,	4
Erysipelas,	1
Total,	54

Total number of prescriptions issued, 317

Many thanks are due to Drs. Wiley and Higby, of the "Sanitarium," for the kind care and attention extended by them to our nurses and infants throughout the hot summer months, which certainly decreased our mortality list to a great extent.

I must also heartily thank our Matron and Assistant (Miss Pearce and Mrs. Parkinson) for the faithful and efficient performance of their duties.

Respectfully submitted,
SARAH A. COHEN, M.D.,
Attending Physician,
822 North Eighth Street.

PHILADELPHIA, January 1st, 1885.

(12)

Contributions.

Atmore, Robt. E.	$10 00	Bailey, Mr. R. H. (Hawthorne, Reading, Pa.)...	$10 00
Ashhurst, Richard L.	25 00	Biddle, Mrs. J. R.	00
A. M. B.	1 00	Bache, Miss Margaret H.	5 00
A Friend	2 00	Buckley, Mrs. Edw. S.	5 00
Aertsen, Mrs James M.	2 00	Blair, Mrs. A. A. (annual).	5 00
A friend of babies.	50	Belfield, Mr. T. Broome.	10 00
A Friend (Manayunk)	20 00	Brown, Mr. Alexander...	50 00
A——, Miss	5 00	"Bertie"	1 00
A Mutual Friend	1 00	Buckley, Mrs. Edw. S.	10 00
A Well-Wisher	75	Birnbaum, Mrs.	3 00
A Friend (through Miss Hattie Trucks)	2 00	Baugh, Mr. Danl.	25 00
A. C. S.	5 00	Biddle, Mrs. Thos. A. (annual)	5 00
Ashhurst, Miss	10 00	
A Friend	25 00	Bar Harbor Entertainment (through Mrs. J. B. Biddle)	600 00
Atmore, Robt. E.	20 00	Brock, Mrs. J. W.	25 00
Ashhurst, Mrs. Richard L.	20 00	
Anonymous (through Mrs. A. A. Blair)	25 00	Clark, E. W. & Co.	25 00
		Campbell, Mrs. St. George.	5 00
A. K. C.	5 00	Converse, Mr. John H.	25 00
Annual Subscription	5 00	C. C.	5 00
A Thank Offering	25 00	Cope, Mrs. John E.	30 00
Anonymous (through Mrs. A. A. Blair)	25 00	Cash	1 00
		Cash	5 00
A Friend (through Miss Harrah)	5 00	Cash	1 00
		Cash	1 00
		Comegys, Miss Anne	2 00
Bonnell, Miss M. A.	1 00	Cash	1 00
Bickley, Mrs. Miriam D.	20 00	Cash	5 00
Burnham, Mr. George	10 00	Cope, Mrs. John E.	15 00
Bunting, Mrs. S. E.	1 00	Childs, Mrs. Isaac R.	5 00
Bunting, Miss	2 00	"Corner Stone"	3 00
Bremer, Mrs.	1 00	Connaroe, Mrs. George	3 00
Biddle, Mrs. Caldwell K.	2 00	Cash	3 75
Biddle, Mrs. John B.	20 00	C. C. B.	1 00
Bliss, Mrs. A. C.	1 00	Coleman, Mrs. E.	5 00
Brown, Mrs. Charlotte A. (Burlington)	50 00	Cope, Mrs. John E.	10 00
		Cadbury, Mr. Joel.	5 00
Bonnell, Mr. H. H.	1 00	C. R. L.	10 00
Bunting, Mrs. S. E.	4 00	Campbell, Mrs. St. George.	5 00
Baugh, Mrs. Danl.	2 00	Coleman, Mrs. Robt. (annual)	25 00
Bache, Mrs. A. D.	2 00	C. C. T.	1 00
Biddle, Mrs. C. K.	2 00	Coffin, Mrs. Lemuel.	10 00
Bartol, Mr. H. W.	15 00	Coates, Mrs. Eliza (annual)	3 00
Bowie, Mrs. Catharine.	5 00	Coates, Mrs. Eliza (extra).	2 00
Buchanan, Rev. Edw. Y.	5 00	Coffin, Mrs. A. G.	25 00
Burnham, Parry, Williams & Co.	50 00	C. E. C.	5 00
Beattie, Mrs. Robt. H.	3 00	Cadbury, Mr. Joel.	5 00
B. T., Mrs.	1 00	Camac, Mr. William.	5 00
Bache, Edith M. Little.	1 00	Cope, Mrs. John E.	10 00
Birnbaum, Mrs. S.	5 00	Carver, Master Willie	1 00

(13)

July 9: I hope I may never see another such time among the children. There is no rest for anyone.

But matters deteriorated futher. As the epidemic peaked, attending physician Emma Boone wearied of the strain and left. Matron Pearce had never favored her, but now, left without medical assistance, the situation seemed hopeless. Then, on July 21, a young, proper-looking doctor arrived at the Sheltering Arms to assume the position of attending physician. Her name was Dr. Sarah Cohen, and she had just turned twenty-six years old.

Though only in her third year of practice, there was much to distinguish Dr. Cohen. A graduate of the Woman's Medical College Class of 1879, she came recommended to the job by Dr. Clara Marshall, professor at the college, who had been instrumental in establishing the Sheltering Arms. Tall and stately, with a deep voice and a self-contained manner, Dr. Cohen lived in the neighborhood, where she shared an office with her two brothers, one a physician and the other a pharmacist. Sarah's own practice consisted of work among the area's immigrant Jewish population, particularly among its women and children, delivering their babies, supervising and prescribing for their illnesses and troubles, and helping to interpret to them their new and difficult lives in America. In coming to the Sheltering Arms, she was extending her own committment, and that of the women's medical movement, to providing health care for needy and deserving women and children.

By mid-August 1883 the measles epidemic had abated. Working without pay, Dr. Cohen gave several hours each day to the home, diagnosing all pediatric illness and prescribing a course of treatment, monitoring the health of the resident mothers, and occasionally advising the Committee on Admissions, Adoption, and Putting Out. Though the home offered "aid and protection to all infants that come, and [did] the work without regard to color, creed, or nationality,"[53] when several of the white wet nurses refused to suckle black infants, Dr. Cohen instructed the staff not to accept any more black babies. The Philadelphia Association for Colored Orphans absorbed some of the foundlings, but did not take children under eighteen months old.

By the end of Dr. Cohen's tenure, and the fourth full year of the home's operation, 223 women and 418 children had been rescued by the Sheltering Arms. Nearly 70 percent of the women had been deemed sufficiently reformed to restore to their children. Another 7 percent of the infants were placed in adoptive families to be raised "as their own."[54]

The Sheltering Arms combined a home setting with medical care and a consciously reforming Christian social posture. It was a formula which its statistics, and the society in which it operated, told them was a great success.

As for Sarah, she remained at the Sheltering Arms as a visiting physician for the next two years, through 1887. Thereafter, she engaged exclusively in private practice. Many years later, a neighbor recalled her as an intimidating woman, one who "had no love in her . . . for anything but medicine. Medicine was what she loved." But in 1883, when Sarah was twenty-six and at the beginning of her career, the staff of the Sheltering Arms had a different reaction. She was, wrote Matron Pearce, "so punctual, so kind, and very nice."[55]

The New England Hospital for Women and Children

Boston, Massachusetts

Among the medical institutions founded by and for women in the nineteenth century, the New England Hospital for Women and Children stands representative of the aims and achievements of the institutional ambitions of the women's medical movement. With the Woman's Medical College of Pennsylvania, the New York Infirmary, and the Chicago Hospital for Women and Children, the New England Hospital for Women and Children created a structure that would treat women and youngsters in need of medical care, educate the female physicians and nurses who would attend them, provide vital clinical and postgraduate experience to women medical students and doctors excluded from clinical privileges at existing male hospitals, and integrate the larger social, moral, and educational aims of the women's medical movement. It did so in an entirely women's sphere, training women students, running the hospital with a female staff, and treating only women patients and their children. Throughout the second half of the nineteenth century, the New England Hospital dominated the region's institutional medical care available to women. Its founders had intended it so from the start.

The New England Hospital was founded by Dr. Marie Zakrzewska, one of the early pioneers in the women's medical movement in America. A native of Germany and European-trained, Zak, as she was known, allied herself in America with doctors Elizabeth and Emily Blackwell and helped in their

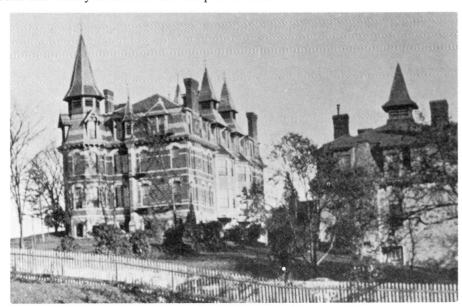

The New England Hospital for Women and Children, Boston (c. 1872). Sophia Smith Collection, Smith College.

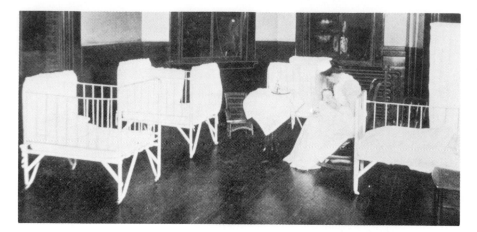

Nurse with child in children's ward, the New England Hospital for Women and Children, Boston (1899). Sophia Smith Collection, Smith College.

Right: *Nurse in operating room at the New England Hospital for Women and Children, Boston.* Sophia Smith Collection, Smith College.

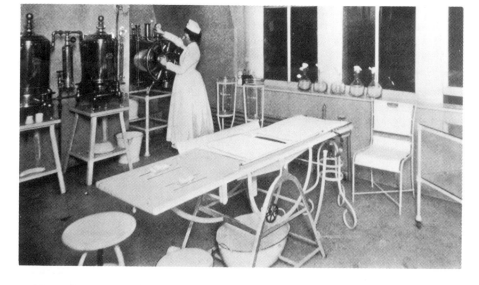

Below: *Nurses at the New England Hospital for Women and Children, Boston (1899).* Sophia Smith Collection, Smith College.

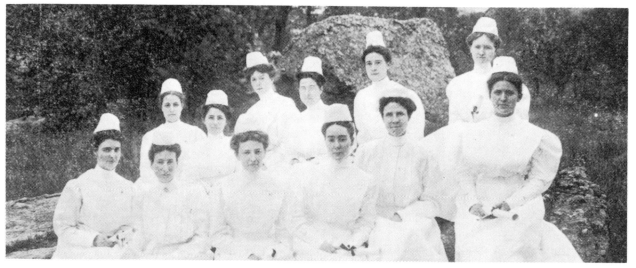

efforts to establish the New York Infirmary. Drawn to Boston by an offer to work with Dr. Samuel Gregory at the New England Female College, Zak eventually broke with him, and set out to establish her own hospital and training school for women.[56]

The project was incorporated in June of 1862, and on July 1 that same year, the New England Hospital for Women and Children opened "in a sunny, airy house" at 60 Pleasant Street in Boston's South End. The institution's aims were

> To provide for women medical aid of competent physicians of their own sex;
> To assist educated women in the practical study of medicine; and
> To train nurses for the sick.[57]

Like other similar institutions before it and to follow, its aims were quickly realized, and by 1864 Zak had to move the hospital to larger quarters on Warren (later Warrenton) Street around the corner. By 1869 the staff was again finding the facilities too small. With funds raised by Zak and the hospital's doctors and directors, enough money was raised to purchase new quarters on a high hill in Roxbury. A towering structure, the hospital attracted patients from across New England and the nation. Throughout the century, half the patients consistently came from counties and regions beyond Boston's borders.[58]

The New England Hospital specialized in obstetrics, pediatrics, and gynecology, but its staff also offered the full range of medical treatment practiced in the nineteenth century, including surgery and outpatient clinics. With specialized programs for diseases of the eyes, ears, nose, and throat; maternity monitoring; and child health clinics, the facility attracted over nineteen thousand patients annually by the end of the century.[59] In Boston, it provided the bulk of maternity care. Boston City Hospital, which opened in 1864, did not establish a gynecological department until 1873, and then only as an outpatient department. Boston Lying-Hospital remained closed between 1856 and 1872. In the 1890s, the New England Hospital was still one of "only seven American hospitals that regularly accepted women."[60]

The New England Hospital was noted for its medical innovation as well as its availability to female patients. Based on her work as chief midwife in Berlin's reknowned Charité Hospital, Zak was among the first doctors in American medicine to introduce sanitary and sterilizing methods during a period when asepsis was still a debate. In 1864, Boston's leading physicians, including Walter Channing, C. P. Rutman, Henry I. Bowditch, and Samuel Cabot signed a circular attesting to the hospital's leadership and successes in preventing contagious fevers at a time when other hospitals could not.[61]

But among the most important services The New England Hospital provided were its clinical training facilities for women physicians. Graduates of the Woman's Medical College of Pennsylvania Class of 1879 pursued pre- and postgraduate training there throughout the 1870s, 80s, and 90s, including 1879 graduates Emma Baldwin, Harriet Belcher, Henrietta Louisa Exton, Sophia Howard, Rachel Nicol, Julia Pease Abbott and Mary Wolfenden Battershall. Their recollections recreate the character both of medical practice at the Hospital and of their own training.

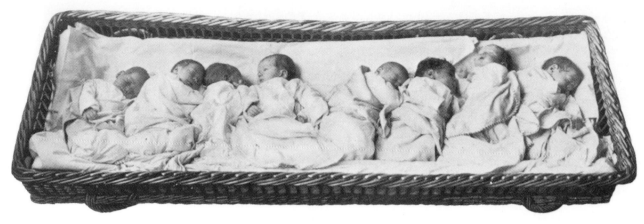

Newborns at the New England Hospital for Women and Children, Boston (1899).
Sophia Smith Collection, Smith College.

Harriet Belcher came to the New England Hospital in 1877.

> I was transferred to the maternity department. Our Resident was dangerously ill with a poisoned wound. Other experienced students were occupied with fever cases. It was unsafe for them to come into my department. I felt I had the world upon my shoulder. Imagine me with eleven babies on my hands at once, to say nothing of their mothers, and of bringing them into the world. This maternity is the saddest of places to me. Most of the women are unmarried, and except for the respectability of the thing, by far the greater number had better not be—the husbands being brutal wretches who abuse them.[62]

In 1879, Belcher's classmate, Rachel Nicol described her experience in the hospital's surgical division:

> I am to spend my first four months in the surgical wards and have already become deeply interested in my patients. Each doctor is expected to visit the patients under her care before breakfast, dinner and supper, also again in the forenoon with the chief of the hospital. After supper each one reports to the chief physician the condition of her patients. Each puts up her own medicines also. Tuesdays and Fridays are set apart from surgical operations.[63]

As for the clinics,

> Clinics are held every morning except Sunday. One of the head doctors comes, sees all the patients in turn, questions, and then prescribes gratuitously, medicine or treatment or both. For which they are able, they pay a trifling sum. On two mornings, clinics begin at 8. We often have between 70 and 80 patients. I have charge of a backroom and give mostly uterine examinations and treatment, but also examine hearts, lungs, bandage, etc. On two other mornings I make up prescriptions in the clinic room, and on the other two can listen or go out to see patients as I choose.[64]

Like the other major women's training and treatment medical institutions, the New England Hospital thrived until the last decade of the nineteenth century. Throughout the 1890s, as many of the women's medical schools and hospitals began to close or merge with male establishments, the New England Hospital kept its doors open. As did the Woman's Medical College of Pennsylvania, it remained committed far into the twentieth century to the exclusive care and education of female patients and doctors. It closed in 1969 as it had begun more than a century before, as an institution designed to serve the special and specific needs of the female medical and patient community. It had provided care and training where once there had been none.

The Highland Home Sanitarium

Cambridgeboro (later Cambridge Springs), Pennsylvania

Almina Rhodes Dean did not apprentice herself to a medical institution in late-nineteenth-century America—she invented one. Alone among the graduates of the Woman's Medical College Class of 1879 who practiced in the United States, she organized a facility for the treatment of medical ills and succeeded in making it one of the most popular curative facilities in her area. Unlike most of her female cohorts who, in the mainstream of the women's medical movement, practiced among women and children, Almina Dean catered to a mixed-sex clientele. In the midst of one of Pennsylvania's most abundant mineral springs resorts and spas, Almina Dean founded the Highland Home Sanitarium, where a traveler or resident could benefit from Dr. Dean's general practice, the area's mineral waters, and the widely lauded "Vacuum Treatment" available exclusively at Dr. Dean's sanitarium.

   Almina Rhodes Dean's career unfolded two miles from where Almina

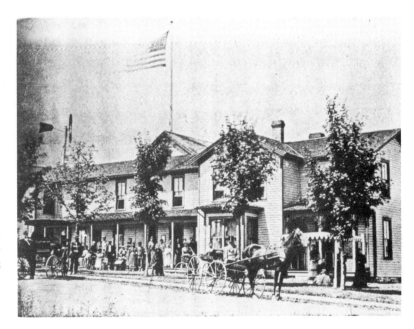

The Highland Home Sanitarium, (c. 1885) Cambridgeboro, Pennsylvania, founded by Dr. Almina Rhodes Dean in 1885. Kreitz Family Collection.

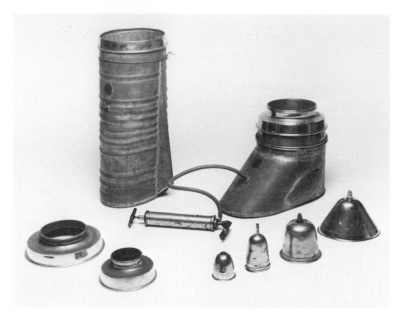

Vacuum used by Dr. Dean. Kreitz Family Collection.

Rhodes had been born on March 16, 1850. Her parents were farmers, who saw to her education at the Edinboro Normal School. An adolescent illness led Almina to take a water treatment at the springs in Danville, New York, and the experience seems to have turned her toward medicine. In the spring semester of 1877, she entered the Woman's Medical College of Pennsylvania, completing her degree in two years. She returned immediately to north central Pennsylvania to set up private practice, and by 1882 she was back in Cambridgeboro, where she built a hospital and home on a tract of land belonging to her family.

The Cambridgeboro Almina Rhodes returned to was a vastly different community from the one into which she had been born. In 1860, the local physician, Dr. John Gray, had drilled a shallow well on his farm in search of oil. The well yielded only water, but Gray would drink from the pool on warm days. Then, in 1884, accompanying a patient to Hot Springs, Arkansas, Gray tried the mineral waters there, and noticed a distinct similarity to the water on his property. Returning to Cambridgeboro, Gray made his spring more presentable, advertised it in the "Cambridge News" as a natural aid for all manner of ills, and began Cambridgeboro's boom as a late-nineteenth-century mineral springs spa.

At its height, Cambridgeboro boasted over fifty hotels and spas, including the Hotel Rider, with its grand lobby "that exceeds in size any other in the world; in it one thousand persons can mingle and be comfortable."[65] Small- and middle-sized institutions abounded as well, and the summer population often trebled the town's resident membership. Into such an enviroment, Almina Rhodes Dean brought her Highland Home Sanitarium, and its success was immediate.

By 1889, when Dr. Dean introduced her "Vacuum Technique," she was already married and the mother of a young daughter. Her husband, a former

HIGHLAND ❈ HOME,

LOCATED AT

The Dale Avenue Mineral Springs,

Cambridgeboro, Crawford County, Pa.,

——On the Line of the N. Y., P. & O. R. R.——

A. P. DEAN, M. D., PHYSICIAN IN CHARGE.

This Institution is designed and specially equipped for the cure of disease by the method known as the

✳ VACUUM TREATMENT, ✳

which is the best remedial agent in chronic diseases known to the medical profession, as has been demonstrated by Dr. Parker, of Chicago, and his predecessors, Drs. Hadfield and Parker, their labors extending over a period of twenty-four years. Paralysis, Locomotor Ataxia, Bright's Disease, Epilepsy, Chronic Rheumatism, Nervous Diseases, Dyspepsia and many other chronic ailments, yield to its judicious use. This treatment is supplemented by Hydropathy, Swedish Movements, Mineral Water, and other hygienic agencies, together with appropriate medication, according to the needs of each patient. For terms address

On notification, Carriage will meet invalids at depot. **M. H. DEAN, Sec.**

Highland Home advertisement (c. 1885). Kreitz Family Collection.

patient in her regular practice and, like her own father, an area farmer, supported his wife's professional efforts. In 1889, she went to Chicago, where she studied "pneumatic medicine," and returned with the Vacuum Equipment that was to become her fame. She purchased a building in town, named it the Highland Home Sanitarium, and thereafter conducted her traditional practice in conjunction with the Vacuum Technique and related mineral waters cure.

The Vacuum Equipment itself consisted of a large metal vacuum pump that attached to various smaller metal forms designed to fit over specific portions of the body. There were forms for arms, legs, breasts—everything but a person's head. The patient would insert the affected body portion into the appropriate form, the vacuum would be turned on, and the pump would suck out the air. The process was repeated several times in succession in an effort to improve circulation and extrude body impurities.

Not a "quack" by any means, Almina Dean was, with her Vacuum Equipment, practicing a contemporary theory of the nature of illness. Her Vacuum Treatment assumed that an imbalance in the body's circulation allowed dangerous poisons to accumulate unnaturally in local areas of the body. Vacuuming the poisons out would restore the necessary balance, in addition to stimulating improved blood flow. In combination with drinking the local healing mineral waters, the waste poisons would be flushed out of the body in efficient form. Her patients continually attested to the success and value of her treatment, and for the rest of her working life, her practice thrived.

Though Almina Dean never practiced in the institutions created specifically to serve the women's medical movement, her career is in many ways typical of those of the women physicians produced by that movement during the second half of the nineteenth century. Her medical treatment supported pure and wholesome living, including a preference for nonalcoholic drugs. Keeping with one of the basic tenets of the women's medical movement—that the natural nurturing powers of women in the home be extended into the community at large—Almina Dean opened up her home to the general population seeking to be healed in it. Her acceptance as a respected physician was reflected in her election in 1885 and 1886 as vice president of the Crawford County Medical Society. Combined with her own belief in the Vacuum Treatment, the medical training she received in the women's medical college system and the skills she acquired there made her one of her area's best-known and most sought-after physicians of her day.

Almina Rhodes Dean died in her home in 1897 of a series of strokes that had left her without speech or easy movement for the year and a half prior. Her death occurred in the year that the citizens of Cambridgeboro formally acknowledged what had made their community, and in large measure Almina Dean's practice, a major nineteenth-century success. With nearly unanimous ballots cast, the town changed its name from Cambridgeboro, Pennsylvania, to Cambridge Springs.

NOTES

1. *Official Report of the Trustees and Officers of the State Hospital for the Insane of Norristown, Pa.,* from September 30, 1881, to September 30, 1882. "Third Report of Trustees" (Allentown, PA: 1882), 5–6.
2. Ibid., 9, 7.
3. Ibid., 24.
4. Ibid., 24–25.
5. Ibid., 9.
6. Ibid., 31.
7. Ibid., 49–50.
8. Ibid., 38–39.
9. Ibid., 26.
10. Ibid., 37, and 35–36.
11. Ibid., 37.
12. Ibid., 39.
13. Ibid., 39.
14. Ibid., 27–28.
15. Ibid., 41.
16. Ibid., 28.
17. Ibid., 29.
18. Ibid., 47.
19. Ibid., 31.
20. Ibid., 30.
21. Ibid., 29.
22. Ibid., 31.
23. Ibid., 32.
24. "Rules in Relation to the Admission of Children in the Nursery and Child's Hospital," in the *Twenty-Fifty Annual Report of the Nursery and Child's Hospital,* March 1st, 1880, (New York: 1880), 86–87.
25. *Twenty-Sixth Annual Report,* 5.
26. Ibid., 20.
27. Ibid., 18.

28. *Twenty-Eighth Annual Report of the Nursery and Child's Hospital* (New York: 1882).
29. *Twenty-Sixth Annual Report,* 6.
30. *Twenty-Sixth Annual Report of the Nursery and Child's Hospital* (New York: 1881).
31. *Twenty-Sixth Annual Report,* 19.
32. Ibid., 6–7.
33. Ibid., 8.
34. *Mary Thompson Hospital: A Report, 1979–1980* (Chicago: 1980), 3.
35. *Nineteenth Annual Report of the Chicago Hospital for Women and Children* (Chicago: 1884), 6–7.
36. Ibid.
37. *Nineteenth Annual Report,* 5.
38. Ibid., 8.
39. Ibid., 10–13.
40. *Sixteenth Annual Report of the Chicago Hospital for Women and Children* (Chicago: 1881), 5.
41. Ibid., 12.
42. A. T. Andreas, *History of Chicago in Three Volumes* (Chicago: 1886), vol. III, *From the Fire of 1871 until 1885,* 520.
43. In 1879 the college moved to its own building at 335–39 South Lincoln Street opposite Cook County Hospital and changed its name to the Woman's Medical College of Chicago. In 1891 it became part of Northwestern University.
44. *Mary Thompson Hospital,* 9, 11.
45. *Report of the Sheltering Arms of the Protestant Episcopal Church in the City of Philadelphia, for 1885* (Philadelphia: 1885), 7.
46. *Report of the Sheltering Arms of the Protestant Episcopal Chruch in the City of Philadelphia: November 1882* (Philadelphia: 1882), 5.
47. Ibid., 7.
48. Ibid., 11.
49. Ibid.
50. Ibid.
51. *Report of the Sheltering Arms . . . 1885,* 12.
52. S. C. Pcarce, *Diary,* The Sheltering Arms, June 1883–January 1887. Entries for June, July, and August 1883. Urban Archives, Temple University.
53. *Report of the Sheltering Arms . . . 1882,* 11.
54. Ruth J. Abram, "Honorable in the Sight of God." Unpublished biography of Sarah Cohen (n.d.), 1.
55. Ibid., 41.
56. On the founding of the New England Hospital for Women and Children, see Virginia G. Drachman, *Hospital with a Heart: Women Doctors and the Paradox of Separatism at the New England Hospital, 1862–1969.* Ithaca, N.Y.: Cornell Univ. Press, 1984; Mary Roth Walsh, *"Doctors Wanted: No Women Need Apply": Sexual Barriers in the Medical Profession, 1835–1975* (New Haven, CT: Yale University Press, 1977); and Ruth J. Abram, "Will There Be a Monument?" in this volume.
57. Agnes C. Victor, ed., *A Woman's Quest: The Life of Marie E. Zakrzewska, M.D.* New York, 1924.
58. Drachman, *Hospital with a Heart,* 64.
59. Walsh, *"Doctors Wanted,"* 96.
60. Ibid., 92–221; Drachman, *Hospital with a Heart,* 61.
61. Walsh, *"Doctors Wanted,"* 93.

62. Letter of Harriet Belcher, September 23, 1877, in the private collection of Alice McCone.
63. Letter of Rachel Nicol, May 16, 1879, in the collection of Pi Beta Phi Sorority, Kansas City, Missouri.
64. Letter of Harriet Belcher, January 20, 1878, in the private collection of Alice McCone.
65. Chuck Stone, ed. *Cambridge Springs Centennial.* Cambridge Springs, Pennsylvania (n.d.). "Early History—Cambridgeboro," no pagination.

Medical Missionaries

"Ourselves Your Servants for Jesus' Sake"

ELLEN J. SMITH

In all, eight of our graduates have engaged in [medical missionary] work in Asia.
—Dr. Rachel Bodley, Dean
Survey of the Living Graduates of the Woman's
Medical College of Pennsylvania, 1881

Members of the Class of 1879 Who Became Medical Missionaries

Dr. Ann S. Kugler

Ten thousand miles separate Ardmore, Pennsylvania, from Guntur, India, but the life and work of Dr. Anna Kugler brought together the thrusts of nineteenth-century women's medical work and evangelical culture in one of the most remarkable careers of the Woman's Medical College Class of 1879.

Born April 19, 1856, Kugler was raised in a Lutheran household that stressed public service and religious dedication. Her father, active in Lutheran lay organizations, served for two years in the Pennsylvania state legislature and helped to establish the first public school in the county. Anna's mother organized the home, raising six children and guiding religious instruction. Anna scarcely recalled a time when religion was not her calling in life, but the visit

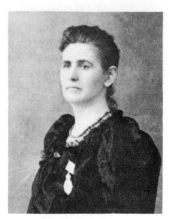

Dr. Anna S. Kugler, wearing medal awarded to her by the Government of India in honor of her service to the people of India (1917). Lutheran Church in America.

to her church by a Baptist missionary from India when Anna was still a girl focused the nature of that calling. The story is told that Anna, returning from the lecture, said simply, "I'll go."[1]

Encouraged by her family, Anna entered the Woman's Medical College of Pennsylvania at age nineteen, graduating with honors with the Class of 1879. As a student she had lived and practiced for several months among Philadelphia's poor. She completed her studies in a postgraduate internship at the Woman's Hospital of Philadelphia, and in 1880 was appointed first assistant physician of the State Asylum for the Insane in Norristown, Pennsylvania, becoming one of the first women in the country to hold such a post. But her desire to be a missionary physician prevailed, and in 1882 she applied to the Lutheran Board of Foreign Missions to be sent abroad.

The executive board of the Women's Missionary Society was, in 1882, still reluctant to sponsor medical work, but agreed to send Kugler to India as a missionary teacher. Praying that God would send her "patients instead of scholars,"[2] Kugler sailed from Philadelphia on August 25, 1883. In her possession was one hundred dollars, plus a hundred-dollar gift from Society of Friends member Rebecca White, which Kugler used to purchase medicines and medical instruments in London. She docked in Madras, India, in early November, and boarded a barge for the 230 mile, thirteen-day trip up the Buckingham Canal to Guntur.[3] On November 28, Kugler was greeted for the first time by the people among whom she was to make her home for the next forty-seven years. The Christian converts among them read Bible verses to her, sang hymns in their native Telegu, and answered the missionaries' questions so well as "to shame some who have had more advantages."[4]

Kugler's career as a missionary teacher, doctor, and friend began immediately. For two years she instructed Hindu and Moslem girls in the mission school, teaching them language, Bible, and hygiene. "We do not change the food, dress or habits of life of these girls, except when necessary to do so for the sake of morality or health," she explained later.[5] Kugler instructed her pupils through the use of scrapbooks and pictures her American friends compiled for her from popular magazines.[6] She likewise brought her missionary teaching to Indian women in her own home and in the natives' houses and villages.

Simultaneously, Kugler began to practice medicine among the women and children of the area's eighteen thousand Europeans, Eurasians, native Christians, Hindus, Moslems, and Parsis. "The young doctor," she wrote of herself,

> had come from a large state hospital, where she had been associated with other physicians as colleagues and consultants, with every facility for becoming a specialist in mental diseases, and from a city noted for its medical schools and hospitals. She was now in the midst of twenty million Telugus, for whom as yet no hospital for women had been built.[7]

Shocked at the condition in which she found Indian women and aware that they would not seek out European medicine in the male-staffed government dispensaries, Kugler determined to provide medical services specifically to women and children. "The *condition* of the women in India is an argument for woman's work . . . ," she wrote in 1887:

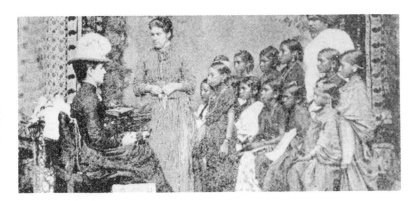

Dr. Anna Kugler, seated, handing out prizes in one of many girls' schools that she founded in India (c. 1884). Lutheran Church in America.

> Ignorant, superstitious, caste-bound, the slave of man's passions, the victim of child-marriage and enforced widowhood—*this* is the condition of the vast majority of the women of India. . . . Only by the elevation of her mothers and daughters can India hope to attain to the heights of true civilizations; that civilization which recognizes woman as an equal not an inferior.[8]

In her first year, she treated 276 patients on the veranda of her porch and 185 patients in their homes. "Patients have been brought to me from villages 12, 20, and 30 miles distant," she recorded. "Though I have repeatedly told them how impossible it was for me to give them the attention they could receive in the government hospital, they invariably preferred to receive what I could give them, because I was a woman."[9]

Kugler moved sensitively among her Indian neighbors and patients. As a foreigner and a Christian, she was initially unable to make direct contact with the Brahmin-caste Hindus. When she visited their houses, she would see patients outdoors, so she would not defile their homes. She placed medicine bottles on the ground rather than give them directly to the patients, "knowing nothing but earth could make them fit to be handled by the ceremonially clean hand of a Brahmin."[10] Eventually, however, supported by leading Hindu families, Kugler became a welcome guest in homes normally barred to Westerners.

But Kugler's abilities as a missionary doctor were severely hampered by the lack of a hospital in the Guntur area. In 1884 she resolved in her diary "to have a hospital within the next two years." A note added later records, "Little did I know of the long years of waiting ahead."[11] By late 1884, her medicines exhausted and no funds coming from either the local mission or America, Kugler suspended her medical activities and immersed herself in the study of Telegu.

But Kugler's fortunes changed dramatically in 1885. Responding to an appeal from the Guntur mission, the Lutheran Women's Missionary Convention in America authorized collection of funds for a woman's hospital and dispensary. In December, Kugler was formally appointed a medical missionary, relieved of her mission teaching duties, and sent $50 for medicines and the rental of a temporary dispensary. Added to the $333 raised among the missionaries themselves, Kugler procured a house in the Moslem section of Guntur, which served as "the first [dispensary] rented in the Telegu country

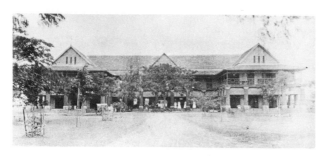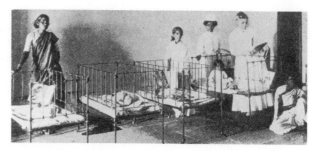

Left: *Guntur Hospital for Women and Children, Guntur, India (1890s).* Lutheran Church in America. Right: *Dr. Anna Kugler making rounds in the Children's Ward, Guntur Hospital for Women and Children, Guntur, India (1890s).* Lutheran Church in America.

for medical work for women."[12] In its first years, the dispensary treated over five thousand patients.

In 1889, Kugler took her first furlough, touring America to raise money and interest in the Guntur mission and its hospital project. She also found time to acquire additional postgraduate medical training. She returned to America again in 1893 to lecture and raise funds, returning via Vienna for brief medical study there. In 1893, on eighteen acres purchased in the north end of town, the Guntur missions's first medical building for women patients was opened—a dispensary—followed in 1895 by a residence for medical missionaries. On January 1, 1897, the long-desired Guntur Hospital, known to the natives as "Yesus Christus," was dedicated, but due to Kugler's ill health and her absence on furlough, the hospital did not begin accepting patients until December 1898.

Opened initially with fifty beds, the Guntur Hospital outgrew its facilities within the first five years, and the complex expanded. In Kugler's lifetime, the medical compound gained a diet kitchen and laboratory annex (1907); a chapel (1909); a children's ward (1911); a training school and home for nurses (1912); a "choultry," or inn for relatives of patients, donated by the Rajah of Ellore (1914); maternity and surgical blocks (1915); and additional smaller buildings. Behind these façades overlooking Victorian lawns, the staff saw over one hundred thousand patients in the dispensary, performed almost eight thousand operations, and delivered over fifteen hundred children each year.[13]

As the medical complex expanded, so too did the medical staff. Until 1884, Kugler managed with no regular assistant. In that year she was joined by an American missionary nurse, Katherine Fahs, who, five years later, opened the mission's nursing school to train native nurses and midwives. Dr. Mary Baer, the second physician to join the staff, arrived in 1895. Other American women doctors and nurses continued to join the mission, as did Indian physicians and nurses. The first female Indian physician, Dr. P. Paru, worked with Kugler from 1911 to 1923, when she returned to her home on the Malabar coast to open a hospital of her own.

But for all of Kugler's medical successes, her main focus remained religious. In her medical hospital work, as in each aspect of her life, Kugler viewed her medical activity as an opportunity for advancing the word of God. A medical missionary, she felt, "finds an avenue to the hearts of those who have hitherto steeled themselves against the missionary."[14] "The ideal medical missionary is one who being thoroughly equipped medically . . . has dedicated that equipment and that enthusiasm to the service of Christ to be used in winning souls for Him."[15]

Kugler's daily schedule and the way she organized the Guntur Hospital complex reflect her belief that the medical missionary should attach "as much importance to the religious teaching as to any part of the day's routine."[16] Rising before dawn, she would receive the night superintendent's report, and then spend an hour in private meditation before attending chapel. An early breakfast was followed by morning rounds, examining patients, prescribing medicines, and attending to her correspondence, accounts, and reports as time allowed.

Surgery was performed one morning per week, with the entire staff made available to assist. Kugler also aided in the training of her nurses, whom she educated to become competent midwives, and in providing religious instruction to her patients and staff. Then followed "breakfast," the midday meal, and a rest hour, which Kugler often spent reading or studying. At three o'clock she began her afternoon rounds, followed by tea and conferences with her nursing staff. Private patients called after tea and far into the evening, usually patients from the upper classes of Indian Hindu and Moslem society. An evening meal was followed by an hour of private devotion, but emergencies and late-arriving patients often kept her up into the night. Her diary indicates that except for private appointments, which were not made on the Sabbath, her schedule went week-round.

As her own days were infused with Christian devotion and education, so, too, were those of her staff, patients, and their relatives. "Bible women" staffed the dispensary waiting room for several hours each day, conducting services and educating patients and visitors in the Gospel. In the hospital, services were conducted for employees, friends, and relatives of the patients, and Bible women ministered to the sick as surely as did the medical staff. Classes were conducted for women and children in the chapel's Sunday School, and a Book Depot made religious literature available to all comers at a nominal fee. A visitor to Guntur recalled Kugler's habit of infusing even routine matters with a religious message. In one case, Kugler had been given permission to enter the private room of a Hindu *rani* (princess). Dr. Kugler picked up her baby, saying, "You know, *Rani,* this is a *Yesu Christu* baby, for it was born in a *Yesu Christu* hospital. You will never teach it to worship idols, will you?"[17] The hospital's motto was "Ourselves your servants for Jesus' sake," and no phrase more aptly summarized the private mission of Anna Kugler, or the evangelical medical culture of America that shaped her forty-seven years of human service in India.

Anna Kugler died in 1930 at age seventy-four, after an illness that had caused her to return to the United States for rest and treatment in the mid-1920s. But she chose to return to India to die, among the people she loved and in the hospital she had founded. In her life she had been honored with the trust and respect of every class and caste of Indian culture. Her work had extended into and beyond the Guntur community. She served on the committee that opened the Interdenominational Union Mission Tuberculosis Sanitarium and served for a time as its acting physician-in-chief. With her close friend Dr. Ida Scudder, she helped establish the Medical College for Women

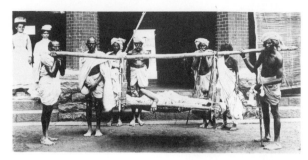

Dr. Anna Kugler in the early 1920s. Lutheran Church in America.

in Vellore, South India, in 1917. The colonial government of Great Britain had awarded her the Kaisar-I-Hind medal in 1905, and the bar to the medal in 1917, the highest honor accorded a non-British subject in India. At her death, thousands mourned her in four separate religious services honoring her memory. She was buried near two other missionary doctors in the cemetery of the hospital that now bears her name.

Eulogizing Kugler, an Indian official observed that "during her life on earth she did not rest for a minute, and all her life was spent in doing good."[18] But Kugler had always observed of herself, "I did nothing. Christ did it all."[19]

NOTES

1. Mrs. Charles P. Wiles, "A Pioneer Medical Missionary: Anna S. Kugler, M.D.," *Lutheran Women* 2 (1961) Philadelphia: Women's Missionary Society of United Lutheran Church of America.
2. William A. Dudde, ed., "100 Years Later: Remembering Anna S. Kugler," *World Encounter* 21 (Fall 1983): 2.
3. Madras, India, is located approximately two hundred miles north of Madras.
4. Dudde, "100 Years Later," 2.
5. Kugler, letter to the General Convention of the Women's Home and Foreign Mission Society, June 1889; Lutheran Church in America Archives, Chicago.
6. Kugler to Mrs. Charles Weiser, January 19, 1884; Lutheran Church in America Archives, Chicago.
7. Margaret R. Seebach, " 'Indian Goddess': The Story of Anna S. Kugler, M.D.," pamphlet published by the Student Volunteer Movement of the International Committee of the Young Men's Christian Association 1942, 2; Lutheran Church in America Archives, Chicago.
8. Kugler, letter to the General Convention of the Women's Home and Foreign Mission Society, April 1887; Lutheran Church in America Archives, Chicago.
9. Dudde, "100 Years Later,": 3.
10. Ibid.
11. Wiles, "A Pioneer Medical Missionary: Anna S. Kugler, M.D.," p. 4.
12. Seebach, " 'Indian Goddess,' " 3.
13. Wiles, "A Pioneer Medical Missionary," 8.
14. Kugler to the General Convention of the Women's Home and Foreign Mission Society, June 1889; Lutheran Church in America Archives, Chicago.
15. Kugler, "Some Problems in Medical Mission Work," date and publisher unknown; Lutheran Church in America Archives, Chicago.
16. Ibid.
17. Seebach, " 'Indian Goddess,' " 5.
18. Ibid., 7.
19. 6.

Medical Societies

"Lifted from the Ranks of Mere Pretenders"

ELLEN J. SMITH

> *The seventh question is the inquiry which, in later years, has assumed with us especial interest in deciding the professional status of women physicians, viz., that of membership in medical societies. Sixty-eight [of the respondents] reply affirmatively to this question. . . .* —Dr. Rachel Bodley, Dean
> Survey of the Living Graduates, of the Woman's
> Medical College of Pennsylvania, 1881

Members of the Class of '79 Who Joined Medical Societies

Avery: Maine Medical Association
Belcher: Rhode Island Medical Association
Dunn (Corey): Connecticut Medical Society, Waterbury Medical Association, Southern California Medical Society, San Diego County Medical Association, Marion County Medical Society, American Medical Association
Flagler: Lycoming County Medical Society
Galt (Simmons): Florida Medical Association, Dade County Medical Association
Howard: Medical Society of the State of New York, Medical Society of the County of Cayuga

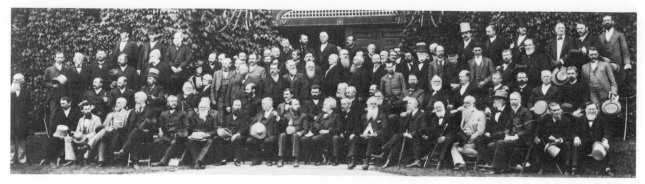

House of delegates to the American Medical Association, Newport, Rhode Island (1889).
Archives, American Medical Association.

Kemp: Dauphin County Medical Society
Presley: Camden County Medical Society, Camden City Medical & Surigcal
          Society, Camden City Medical Society (Secretary), American Med-
          ical Association
Rhodes (Dean): Crawford County Medical Society (vice president, 1885–86)
Richardson: County Medical Society, American Medical Association
Weaver (Soule): Rhode Island Medical Society
Wolfenden (Battershall): Attleboro Doctor's Club, Massachusetts Medical
          Society
Fitch Wood: Courtland Medical Society

Medical societies in the late ninteenth century, as Rachel Bodley observed,
did help to decide the professional status of women physicians. The graduates
of the Class of 1879, with other women physicians of their generation, anticipated becoming members of the various local, state, and national medical
societies that gained in membership, status, and prestige over the course of
the latter nineteenth century. It was in medical societies that physicians could
meet to exchange information on medical ideas, techniques, and innovations.
American medical societies were involved with medical licensing, setting
professional standards, establishing fees, controlling schedules, and generally
standardizing their profession. Through medical societies, physicians received
case referrals and recommendations to hospital and other professional appointments. Indeed, by the late nineteenth century, medical society membership was a virtual prerequisite for most hospital affiliation. Perhaps most
important, medical societies provided one of the few means for separating
the rising self-conscious body of regular physicians from irregular practitioners, and publicly distinguishing "qualified" physicians from the lay doctors,
charlatans, and quacks. Membership in medical societies accorded its members status, economic and professional advantage, and consciously sought to
establish "inside" and "outside" groups within the profession.

    Entrance to medical societies was, from their inception, competitive.[1]
Physicians generally needed to pass an entrance examination, submit letters
of reference from current society members and other professional physicians
with whom they had worked or studied, and finally be voted into admittance
by an executive committee, and ultimately the entire society membership.

Over the course of the nineteenth century, membership in medical societies rose steadily, and by 1900, some 30 percent of male physicians recorded medical society affiliation.[2]

Women physicians recorded substantial society membership as well. But as women's access to male medical schools and hospital training programs was often limited in the late nineteenth century, so too was women doctor's access to male medical societies. Women therefore founded and generally joined all-women's groups they established for themselves, not to compete but to run parallel to the male medical societies upon which they were modeled. As was their goal with medical education, so too was it in professional affiliation—to be admitted freely and incorporated into the proceedings of integrated medical societies.

The first women physician to seek admission to a state medical society was Dr. Nancy Talbot Clark of Boston, in 1852. Supported in her bid before the Massachusetts Medical Society by Henry Bowditch, she wrote, "I ask this in order that, thereby, I may be publicly lifted from the rank of mere pretender to learning."[3] Though no by-laws specifically prohibited the admission of women candidates, the Society voted against Clark's petition, and refused to accept application from women physicians for the next twenty years. In 1873, the Massachusetts Medical Society heard the petition of Dr. Susan Dimock, but rejected it after long debate. Not until 1884 did the Massachusetts Medical Society finally admit a woman, accepting the application of Dr. Emma Call of the New England Hospital for Women and Children.

Not all state medical societies, however, were as reluctant as the Massachusetts one to accept female physicians. In 1877, Kansas, Rhode Island, and Michigan opened their state medical societies to women.[4] By 1881, seventeen state societies accepted women as members.[5] In Rhode Island, Dr. Harriet Belcher enjoyed a warm reception within the local medical community: "The professional brethren whom I met, far from looking askance at me . . . welcomed me, spoke of my joining their societies at once, told me to use their names as references in obtaining board. One drove me out to persuade his mother to take me in."[6] Dean Rachel Bodley of the Woman's Medical

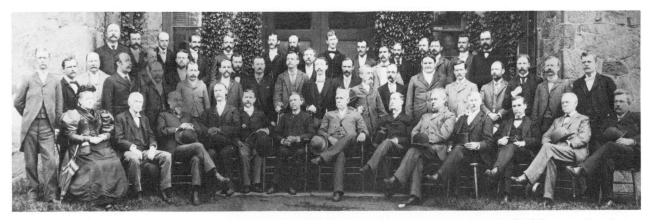

Dr. Sophia Presley and members of the Camden County Medical Society, New Jersey (1869). Camden County Medical Society.

College of Pennsylvania wrote congratulating Dr. Agnes Kemp on her admission in 1880 to the Dauphin County [Pennsylvania] Medical Society. "My dear friend," she began,

> I . . . rejoiced to read in the Public Ledger of June 5th [1880] . . . that at the last regular meeting of the Dauphin County Medical Society, you were admitted as a member of its body. I hasten to offer my congratulations on this auspicious event and to express the hope that you will prove a valuable member.
> . . . Let me hear from your successes from time to time and come see us when you can. You are one in whose career we are greatly interested.[7]

Other women in the Woman's Medical College Class of 1879 broke sexual barriers in their local medical societies as well. In May 1890, Dr. Sophia Presley became the first woman admitted to the Camden County [New Jersey] Medical Society, some seven years after her initial application for admission. The Society's minutes record, "Dr. Sophia Presley, a graudate of the Woman's Medical College of 1879 was elected a member. This was the first female physician ever elected to a membership in this Society. Dr. Presley applied for the admission to the Society in 1883, but the application was postponed for several years and then dropped."[8] Among thc Class of 1879, thirteen of its twenty graduates successfully joined regular male/mixed-sex medical societies. Dr. Almina Rhodes (Dean) eventually served as vice president (1885–86) of the Crawford County [Pennsylvania] Medical Society. Records list her as a dues-paying member beginning in 1880, the year after she graduated from medical school. Other Woman's Medical College graduates belonged to medical societies in Maine, Massachusetts, Connecticut, Rhode Island, New York, New Jersey, Pennsylvania, Florida, Ohio, and California.

But despite the very real inroads women physicians made into medical societies toward the end of the nineteenth century, not enough women were accepted or fully integrated into the societies that did admit them to satisfy the women's medical community. Medical societies specifically excluding women proliferated in this period; in the first seventy-five years of participation in the Massachusetts Medical Society, only one woman was invited to give the annual oration.[9] Though their goal was always integration into the mainstream of American medicine and medical institutions, women found it necessary to create female alliances and organizations that would keep them abreast of medical issues, involve them in collegial groups, and afford them the professional status and visibility that professional affiliation awarded, but from which they were often excluded.

Women's medical societies, as had women's medical colleges before them, arose as parallel institutions to men's, designed to serve many of the same functions. The first women's medical society in the United States was formed in Boston in 1878 by twelve women physicians, most of whom were associated with the New England Hospital for Women and Children.[10] The Woman's Medical College Alumnae Association, formed in 1875, served the function of a national women's medical society for years after its founding. The organization's aim, as stated in its constitution, was threefold.

—The advancement of women in the study of medicine and their due recognition in the practice thereof throughout the country;

The Practitioner's Society (later the Blackwell Society) of Rochester, New York (1890s). Edward G. Miner Library, Rochester, New York.

—Their mutual interest and benefit, and the cultivation of friendly feeling among the alumnae;

—The encouragement of its members in regular practice, according to the code of ethics of the American Medical Association.[11]

Annual meetings of the association included organizational business, the reading of papers on medical subjects, reports of cases, discussion of medical topics, and the ongoing work and reports of various standing committees. "The object of this Association is to stimulate the flagging interest in the discussion of medical subjects among medical women," its president noted, continuing, "The very object of the Association is to offer a reason to medical women for writing; to urge the members of this Association to write, or rather to study, some subject so thoroughly that they shall have something to say about it."[12] The organization's *Proceedings* were published regularly in the report of its annual meetings and distributed throughout the country to its membership.

But though the stated aims of the alumnae association were parallel to those of male medical societies, the content of its proceedings was quite different. Medical reports, discussions of cases, and papers read before the membership tended to reflect health concerns in the women's medical sphere: pediatric, obstetric, and gynecological cases; public health and sanitation issues; and topics relating to diet, exercise, and women's dress. The *Report of Proceedings of the Annual Meeting* of March 1880, for example, included papers on the following subjects: "Case of Removal of Both Ovaries, for the Relief of a Fibroid Tumor of the Uterus" (Dr. Anita Tyng); "Case of Ovariotomy" and "Sarcoma of the Uterus" (Dr. Charlotte Brown); "Reports of Two Cases of Periuterine Cellulitis" (Dr. Harriet A. Bottsford); "Case of Pelvic Maematocele—Subperitoneal" (Dr. Elizabeth J. Holcombe); as well as more general reports on medicine in Utah, autopsies for heart disease, and treatment of ventral hernias. A decade later, the *Report* for 1890 included such articles as "Tenement Houses in Philadelphia" (Dr. Frances Van Gasken); "Some Suggestions from a Case of Malaria Complicating Pregnancy" (Dr. Ada R. Thomas); and "The Correction of Rotary Lateral Curvature of the Spine by Means of Gymnastics—Minus Apparatus" (Dr. Bertha Lewis),

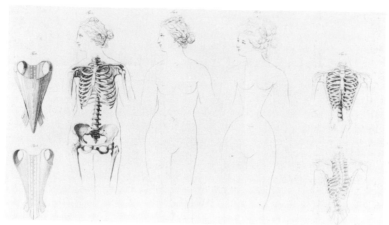

I!lustration of the damage done to the body structure by corsets (1973). NLM.

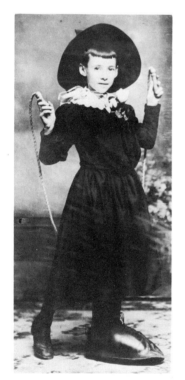

Child with deformed foot holding jumprope. Burns archive.

in which Lewis reported, "My first step was to convince her of the imperative necessity of giving up her corset."[13]

Throughout the last decades of the ninteenth century, the focus of physicians on issues relating to female health continued to be reflected in their professional exchanges. As the century drew to a close, women physicians seemed to pay particular attention to new views of exercise, and especially its benefits to women, topics rarely reported in the proceedings of male medical societies.

"Last spring, I had a patient with pelvic trouble," Dr. Werner reported in 1889, "who after a course of 'rest' treatment was advised to take out-door exercise. She took to bicycle riding, and within the past two weeks has developed into a round, healthy, robust woman. Before that she was pale and sallow."[14] Dr. Ladd reported, "I believe that girls can jump rope occasionally without bad effects, but the lower extremities get more exercise than the upper ones anyhow, and therefore, I advocate the arm movements."[15] Dr. Schneider (Blum) asked, "Does walking increase the menstrual flow? I know of one case where walking was practiced in order to reduce it without any effect upon the menstrual flow."[16]

Women's medical societies, as did their male counterparts, also spent time guarding against inroads made into their profession by "irregular" practitioners. Dr. Elizabeth Keller, president of the Woman's Medical College Alumnae Association, raised the issue at the 1885 meeting: "Dr. Charlotte M. Fay was reported as practicing homeopathy. I wrote Dr. Fay who replied that she was a true homeopathist. Therefore, I move, in accordance with the constitution and by-laws of the Association, that the name of Dr. Fay be dropped from the roll of membership."[17]

What actually constituted an "irregular" practitioner was also a subject of debate in the societies. Dr. Clara Marshall, on the faculty of the Woman's Medical College, raised the issue in 1881, asking, "What constitutes irregular practice? Are we at liberty to get information anywhere and to use it? For instance, water treatment?"[18] Dr. Victoria Scott reported favorably on electrical galvanization to the association in 1885. "In my experience, only one case that had been treated with electricity required operation," she observed,

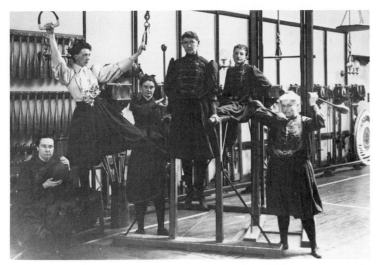 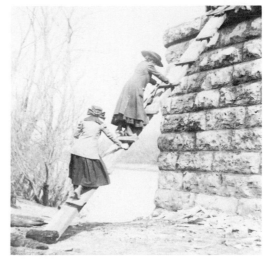

Left: *Women in Gym (1893)*. The Staten Island Historical Society; photograph by Alice Austen. Right: *Women hikers climbing bridge (c. 1905)*. Minnesota Historical Society.

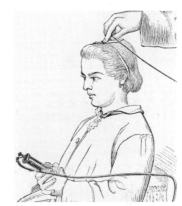

"Fibroids, inflammations, hemorrhages, etc. are all relieved by electricity."[19]

Nineteenth-century medical societies did, then, serve the many functions asked of them by American physicians. From information clearing-houses to organizations designed to define and ultimately protect the profession they represented, medical societies proved to be a strong statement by the medical profession about the role and character of medical practice in the United States. In the overall aims for such organizations, men and women physicians shared a common view. But in the evolution of separate and parallel organizations for male and female practitioners, and in the different nature of issues raised by the two groups, the structure of professional associations spoke of the special and separate sphere assumed for nineteenth-century women's medicine.

Illustration of central galvanization (1881).

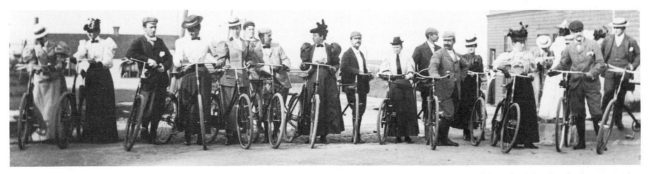

Staten Island Bicycle Club Tea (1895). The Staten Island Historical Society; photography by Alice Austen.

NOTES

1. The first medical society was founded in New Jersey, in 1766. Others followed, including the national American Medical Association in 1846, but not even the AMA attracted members in large numbers until the late nineteenth century. In 1901, the American Medical Association reorganized itself as a federation of state societies, and by 1920 AMA claimed a 60 percent membership among licensed physicians. The American Medical Woman's Association was founded in 1915. See Paul Starr, *The Social Transformation of American Medicine: The Rise of a Sovereign Profession and the Making of a Vast Industry* (New York: Basic Books, 1982), 40, 109–110.
2. Starr, *Social Transformation,* 109.
3. Mary Roth Walsh, *"Doctors Wanted: No Women Need Apply": Sexual Barriers in the Medical Profession, 1835–1975* (New Haven, CT: Yale University Press, 1977), xv, 151.
4. Ibid., 155.
5. Ibid., 159.
6. Harriet Belcher to Eliza Johnson, July 13, 1879, Alice McCone Collection.
7. Letter of Rachel Bodley to Agnes Kemp, June 7, 1880, in Nellie Blessing Eyster, *A Noted Mother and Daughter* (San Francisco, Tomoye Press, 1909), Dorothy Lawrence Collection.
8. Camden County Medical Society Minutes, May 1890 entry; Camden County Medical Society. MCP.
9. Walsh, *"Doctors Wanted,"* 213, 263.
10. Ibid., 104.
11. *Constitution and Report of Proceedings of Annual Meeting,* Alumnae Association of the Woman's Medical College of Pennsylvania, March 11, 1880.
12. *Report of Proceedings of the Twentieth Annual Meeting,* Alumnae Association of the Woman's Medical College of Pennsylvania, May 9 and 10, 1895.
13. Ibid., 129.
14. Woman's Medical College Alumnae Association Transactions, February 14, 1890.
15. Ibid.
16. Ibid.
17. Woman's Medical College Alumnae Association Transactions, 1885.
18. Ibid., 1881.
19. Ibid., 1895.

Family and Community Life

Cordial Social Recognition ELLEN J. SMITH

> *The third question relates to the social status of the woman physician in the community in which she dwells.*
>
> *One hundred fifty-seven answer this question, and of these 150 report cordial social recognition. . . .*
>
> *"What influence has the study of medicine had upon your domestic relations as wife and mother?" . . . The answers of the fifty-two married ladies who respond to this question tabulate as follows: Influence, favorable, 45; not entirely favorable, 6; unfavorable, 1.* —Dr. Rachel Bodley, Dean
>
> Survey of the Living Graduates of the Woman's
> Medical College of Pennsylvania, 1881.

Community Involvement of the Class of 1879

Belcher: Rhode Island Women's Club; Sorosis of Newark
Exton: New Jersey Society of the Colonial Dames of America; American
      Society for the Prevention of Cruelty to Animals; American Anti-
      Vivisection Society
Flagler (Hagenbuch): Society of Friends
Galt (Simmons): Housekeepers' Club of Coconut Grove (Florida)

Howard: Woman's Christian Temperance Union
Kemp: Suffrage Association; Woman's Christian Temperance Union; Magdalen Society; Universal Peace Union; kindergarten movement
Kugler: Board of Foreign Missions of the Lutheran Church
Nicol: J. C. Sorosis Society
Pease (Abbott): Ladies' Auxiliary of Lawrence (Massachusetts) General Hospital
Presley: Young Women's Christian Association; Methodist Episcopal Home, Camden (New Jersey)
Weaver (Soule): Rhode Island Women's Club
Wolfenden (Battershall): Massachusetts Republican Club; Woman's Republican Club; woman's suffrage

Postgraduate Marriages of the Class of 1879

Cohen (May): at age 32, 11 years after graduation
Dunn (Corey): at age 36, 9 years after graduation
Flagler (Hagenbuch): at approximately age 48, approximately 7 years after graduation[1]
Galt (Simmons): at age 37, 12 years after graduation
Pease (Abbott): at age 33, 2 years after graduation
Rhodes (Dean): at age 34, 5 years after graduation
Schneider (Blum): at age 28, 3 years after graduation
Weaver (Soule): at age 34, 7 years after graduation
Wolfenden (Battershall): at age 33, 11 years after graduation

Members of the Class of 1879 Who Had Children

Cohen (May): 2
Dunn (Corey): 3
Flagler (Hagenbuch): 1 adopted child
Kemp: 3; 2 died in infancy
Kugler: 1 adopted child
Pease (Abbott): 4; 2 died in infancy
Rhodes (Dean): 1
Schneider (Blum): 1
Weaver (Soule): 2; 1 died in infancy
Wolfenden (Battershall): 1

The nineteenth-century social ethic that ascribed to women special moral insights, nurturing abilities, and responsibilities to educate and raise the younger generations was the same ethic with which most women ventured forth from their homes and into the professional world. Though breaking out of the specifically family-based sphere assigned to Victorian womanhood, professional women, including women physicians, did so by extending the terms of that sphere to the larger world. They generally assumed of themselves what society did: that as physicians, they could combine their scientific and medical interests with their special educative and reforming powers and so extend the exacting responsibilities of Victorian womanhood to society in general. Uniquely able to integrate science and morality, women physicians could contribute toward healing social as well as medical ills. Nineteenth-century women physicians were, in the words of Regina Morantz-Sanchez, the "connecting link" between the science of the medical profession and the everyday life of women and the Victorian family.[2] They were at once clinicians, reformers, mothers, wives, and the moral guides of the varieties of communities they served.

Nineteenth-century women physicians described their own roles in terms of Victorian womanhood. Noting that women were again making successful entrance into the medical profession, Dr. Lucy Weaver (Soule) noted before a meeting of the Rhode Island Women's Club that there were nevertheless many difficulties. Among the chief threats to legitimate women practitioners, she observed, were both the range of irregular practitioners and women who practiced medicine in an "unwomanly" way:

> It is possible for a woman to be a competent physician, and still to keep her full measure of womanliness, but many a noble woman meets with opposition simply because there are so many women, ignorant and incompetent, who attempt to practice medicine, while still others, reliable in their professions, are not womanly.[3]

A "womanly" practice, however, still gave nineteenth-century women doctors great leeway. Their practices tended to revolve around issues of women's health and hygiene; their work included teaching and educating as well as healing. The physicians' commitment to improving the circumstances that promoted health, as well as the individual health of their patients, encouraged many into active political and reform roles. Combined with their private responsibilities as wives and mothers, sisters and daughters, this commitment caused nineteenth-century women physicians to see themselves as people with an almost sacred responsibility, fulfilling the expectations of their families and communities. In doing so, they were extending the nineteenth-century definition of womanhood itself, but in ways, ironically, that nineteenth-century women physicians may not even have perceived.

The Woman's Medical College Class of 1879 graduates present good profiles of how women physicians in the late nineteenth century organized and conducted their family, civic, and professional interests. Of the class's twenty graduates, nine of them, nearly half, married after graduation.[4] Three of the graduates were married before entering the Woman's Medical College. Eight of the Woman's Medical College graduates, again almost half, never married.

Even among those women who remained unmarried, some expected that one day they might. Indeed, they had every reason to believe they might, for although Julia Pease (Abbott) married just two years after graduation, the average age at marriage for the Class of 1879 was thirty-five, and the average number of years between graduation and marriage was seven and a half.[5]

Of the eleven Woman's Medical College graduates in the Class of 1879 who married at some point in their lives, nine are known to have had children, most within a year or two of their marriages. Phoebe Flagler (Hagenbuch), who married for the third time at age forty-eight, seven years after her graduation, adopted a child. (Anna Kugler, a missionary doctor in India who never married, also adopted a child.)

The Class of 1879 graduates who did marry adapted their practices to the wide varieties of lives into which their family situations led them. Sarah Cohen (May), who practiced among Philadelphia's immigrant poor, married a shoe store owner. Eleanor Galt (Simmons) married a lawyer and sometime manufacturer of guava jelly. Several women married farmers and men with rural backgrounds much like their own. Three of the graduates—Julia Pease (Abbott), Lucy Weaver (Soule), and Mary Wolfenden (Battershall)—married physicians. But whatever their marital situations, most of the class's graduates continued their medical careers. Among the three who eventually left their medical work, one, Lucy Weaver (Soule), did so when her husband retired; another, Louise Schneider (Blum), became "lady principal" at her husband's military academy after fifteen years of her own private practice; and a third, Julia Pease (Abbott), helped establish the Lawrence General Hospital in Lawrence, Massachusetts.

Nevertheless, pursuing professional life while running a marriage and family was a complicated affair. Married physicians profited from the fact that most nineteenth-century medical practices were conducted from the physicians' homes. Most of the married women with families conducted their practices in their homes. All retained domestic help. Each, in combining a career with her family life, defined in a new way the possibilities of nineteenth-century womanhood, extending nurturing and moral character to society at large. A closer look at a few of the lives of the 1879 graduates gives insight both as to how they managed and as to how the society in which they lived both encouraged and circumscribed the dual roles they played as family and professional women.

Mary Alice Avery

Mary Alice Avery never married, but in may ways she is typical of the Woman's Medical College Class of 1879 and of the type of woman in general who became a physician in late-nineteenth-century America. Born on Christmas Eve in 1849, on a small farm in Campton, New Hampshire, Mary Alice was second in a family of seven children. The Avery clan was solid New England stock; Mary Alice descended from the great Boston puritan emigrée preacher John Cotton, and her parents' families had made their homes in rural New Hampshire for generations. Mary Alice was educated in a local private academy, taking a full curriculum of languages, sciences, and mathematics. She graduated at age twenty and taught for the next eight years. In 1877 she enrolled in the Woman's Medical College, graduating two years later at age thirty. Her career and connections thereafter intertwined with previous Woman's Medical College graduates and with institutions they had helped establish and then ran.

Mary Alice Avery's first position was with Dr. Elizabeth Keller (Woman's Medical College Class of 1871), formerly of the New England Hospital for Women and Children. Avery joined her in private practice in Boston in 1879.

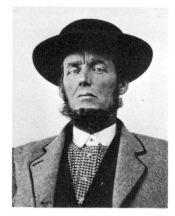

Leonard R. Avery, father of Mary Alice Avery, was a farmer in Campton, New Hampshire. Avery Family Collection.

A year later, Avery began a two-year stint at the Nursery and Child's Hospital, Country Branch, on Staten Island. From 1882 to 1886 she served as assistant physician in the Department for the Insane of the Philadelphia Hospital. There she achieved attention not only for her regular medical abilities, but for a remarkable act of heroism:

> On the night of February 12, 1885, a fire occurred in the Insane Department, resulting in the destruction of the building and the death of sixteen patients by suffocation, the smoke and the heat making it impossible to unlock their doors. . . . There was much noble work done by officials, employees, and firemen in rescuing patients; but the heroic act of the fire was accomplished by Dr. Mary Alice Avery, the Assistant Female Physician. This brave, good woman, accompanied by an epileptic patient, went the entire length of the fourth story, a distance of 800 feet, and rescued a patient who was locked in a room, three sides of which were exposed to the flames. There was no means of escape from this ward except by retracing their steps, and the smoke was so stifling that it was necessary to break windows to prevent suffocation as they stumbled along their perilous way.[6]

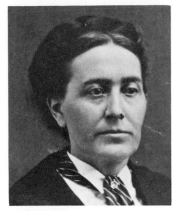

Mary (Cotton) Avery, mother of Mary Alice Avery. Avery Family Collection.

A year later, the hospital offered Dr. Avery the directorship, but she declined, removing instead to Portland, Maine, where she established a private practice in obstetrics, gynecology, pediatrics, and surgery, a practice "larger, in fact, than could well be met without overwork."[7] She died in her sister's home in Lakeport, New Hampshire, in 1904, of an organic heart disease that had afflicted her for several years.

For Mary Alice Avery, her sisters and brothers, their spouses, and her nieces and nephews comprised a loving and extended family to which she was always firmly tied. Her community extended from her cohort of women physicians and teachers from her college years to the variety of institutional and private communities that she served. Her eulogy summarized her many places of belonging, for as a woman and as a physician in late-nineteenth-century America, Dr. Mary Alice Avery had been welcomed and well loved:

> *To how many homes she brought solace and courage;*
> *to how many hearts new life and hope.*[8]

Agnes Nininger Saunders Kemp

The practice of medicine gave most of the graduates of the Woman's Medical Class of 1879, entry into the larger community and both helped define their political activities and professional associations and served as a platform from which they could educate their patients and society at large. The sense that nineteenth-century womanhood possessed special moral qualities and insights encouraged women physicians to extend the "socially transforming aspects of a woman's role in the home"[9] to society in general. This extension of woman's sphere they shared with all women reformers of the nineteenth century, and most alumnae of the Class of 1879 were involved with various reform causes. But no graduate of the Class of 1879 captures the breadth of

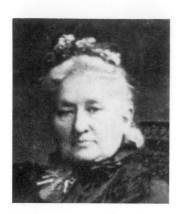

Dr. Agnes Kemp, vice president, Universal Peace Union (c. 1888). Dorothy Lawrence Collection.

interests and energy of these nineteenth-century reformers so well as Agnes Nininger Saunders Kemp.

Kemp's medical degree, coming in her middle age, extended an already established record in reform work and women's rights. An international leader in the temperance movement, Kemp brought the full weight of her scientific and medical training to her religious zeal for pure, holy, and healthy living. In Kemp's career, the connected web of nineteenth-century medicine, reform, and notions of woman's morally transforming responsibilities emerged fully entwined.

Agnes Kemp was born in 1823 in Harrisburg, Pennsylvania, into a deeply committed Quaker family. Only two of her parents' nine children survived infancy, and Mrs. Nininger died when Agnes was a small girl. Her father, a butcher and victualler, educated her, and while still nearly a girl herself, Agnes married her childhood sweetheart, Colonel William Saunders. Illness a few years later prompted Agnes to take a water cure in New York, where she met the nineteenth-century reformers William Lloyd Garrison, Lucretia Mott, Ralph Waldo Emerson, Wendell Phillips, Abbey Kelly Foster, and Elizabeth Peabody.[10] Her entry into their circles encouraged her in her reform efforts in Harrisburg, and Agnes carried out her work with zeal, eventually attracting Lucy Stone (Elizabeth Blackwell's sister-in-law), Julia Ward Howe, and Lucretia Mott[11] to Harrisburg to speak on behalf of their shared reform causes.

Agnes's own special reform interest was temperance, and she was instrumental in establishing the first chapter of the Woman's Christian Temperance Union in Harrisburg. Convinced that temperance reform could only be achieved through universal education, she was an equally strong advocate of the public kindergarten movement, prison reform, defeat of "unholy living," and the Magdalen Society. By her mid-forties, she was a recognized national reform leader.

Widowed early in her first marriage to Colonel Saunders, Agnes married Joseph Kemp in 1857, when she was thirty-seven. Their first two children died in infancy, but in 1860 a daughter, Marie Antoinette, was born, who would become Kemp's lifelong companion and dear friend.

Her second husband's death in 1875 provided Agnes Kemp with an additional focus to her reform activities. Having asked herself how she could now be "the best benefit to my own sex,"[12] she concluded that ignorance of the laws of hygiene sat at the root of most diseases peculiar to women. Convinced of the scientific basis both to rules of hygiene and to the effects of alchohol on the body's organs and functions, Kemp entered the Woman's Medical College of Pennsylvania to take her medical degree. She graduated in 1879, the same year that her daughter, Marie, graduated as valedictorian of her class from Swarthmore College. When she received her medical degree at age fifty-six, Agnes Kemp was the oldest member of the Class of 1879.

Kemp immediately set up private practice in her hometown of Harrisburg and brought her new abilities to bear on her interests in education and reform. In 1880 she was admitted as the first female member of her county's medical society. But her temperance work remained paramount, and in 1887, she and Marie sailed for Europe. They spent the winter of 1887 studying medicine and language respectively at the University of Zurich, and the next two winters in Paris at the Sorbonne and College de France. In Paris, Kemp received her greatest audiences and fame for her temperance reform campaigns, giving such lectures as "Health and Physical Culture," "Social Purity," and "Temperance."[13] The *New York Tribune* reported of her success, "Mrs. Agnes Kemp, a Harrisburg woman, electrifies a Parisian audience by her eloquence."[14] Her message was consistently simple. Medical science proved what God's law insisted: liquor destroyed humanity; temperance perfected it. The stakes were very high:

> A law suit has been set up in the Supreme Court of Public Opinion, viz.: the women of the nation versus the liquor traffic, and before this question can be settled there is much work to be done intelligently and scientifically—for science is but the unfolding of God's laws.[15]

And the "how" of perfecting society was clear:

> The W.C.T.U. believes that the educational method is one of the surest and shortest ways of reaching the desired end. We believe the people are intemperate from ignorance rather than from choice, and that if the facts relating to the evil effect of alchohol were fully known, the common sense of the community would lead to the most important and lasting benefits to the nation. . . . This knowledge must be imparted to men, women, and children, particularly to the latter. Save our boys and girls now.[16]

Agnes and Marie Kemp returned to the United States in 1891, where Agnes resumed her Harrisburg practice and national lecturing, and Marie took a professorship of German at Swarthmore College. In 1895 Marie married Swarthmore physics professor George Hoadley, and in 1901 their son, Anthony, was born. Agnes retired in 1903 and moved to Swarthmore to live with the Hoadleys; she was there in 1907 when Marie died, leaving Agnes to raise her grandson in her son-in-law's house.

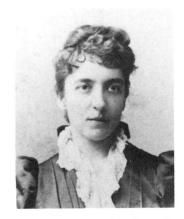

Marie A. Kemp, daughter of Dr. Agnes Kemp, on the day of her graduation from Swarthmore College (c. 1880). Dorothy Lawrence Collection.

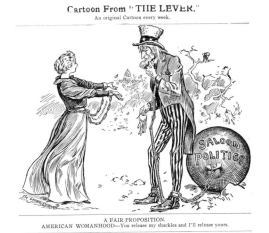

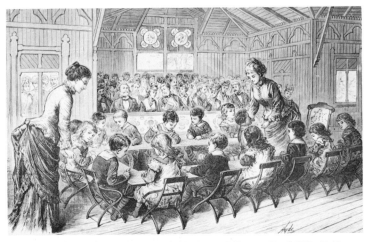

Left: *Prohibition cartoon from the* Chicago Lever. Schlesinger Library, Radcliffe College. Right: *Model kindergarten in Woman's Pavilion, 1876 Centennial, Philadelphia.* Free Library, Philadelphia.

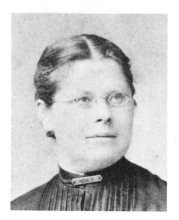

Dr. Louise Schneider Blum (1880s). Petrulias Family Collection.

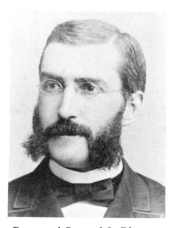

Reverend Samuel J. Blum, husband of Dr. Louise Schneider Blum (1880s). Petrulias Family Collection.

Dr. Agnes Kemp died the following year, in 1908, at age eighty-five. At her request, her body was cremated and her ashes placed next to the grave of her first husband, Colonel William Saunders, in the Harrisburg cemetery. Even in her last year of life, after the death of her daughter, Kemp kept her extraordinary energy and optimism. Delivering a talk entitled "Elixir Vitae" to a gathering of her supporters, she urged, "preserve the happy, joyous *love of life* which is one of the elements of life."[17] Summarizing her own views, and her own career as educator, healer, and believer in the moral strength and reforming powers of womanhood, she concluded, "Knowledge is the fulcrum, intelligence the lever, and courage the power that moves the world."[18]

Louise Schneider Blum

Like Agnes Kemp, Louise Schneider Blum combined medicine, family life, and community service over the course of her adult life. But unlike Kemp, Louise Schneider Blum organized her various roles in a style that marked the distinct stages of her lifetime. After a successful career as a physician, Blum left her practice to help her husband run a boys' school. But she viewed here two careers as of a piece: improving the knowledge and condition of those she served.

Louise was born in Philadelphia in 1854, to Moravian immigrant parents. Educated at the Normal School in Philadelphia, Louise enrolled in the Woman's Medical College in 1876, where she wrote a thesis entitled "Anaesthesia in Natural Labor." She followed her graduation with two years of postgraduate study in Zurich, Switzerland, and in 1881 returned home to take a job in the Woman's Hospital of Philadelphia, serving as surgeon and directing the hospital's free clinics. "She was one of the first women doctors of the city to hold free clinics . . . and did wonderful work in the poorer sections of the city,"[19] her obituary would later relate. It was the start of a medical career that, like those of so many of her graduating cohorts, emphasized health care for women, children, and those without proper access to medical treatment. In late 1882, she opened her own private practice, continuing to work on issues of women's health and hygiene.

Her involvement with the Moravian Church brought her in contact with the Reverend S. J. Blum, pastor of the Fifth Moravian Church in Philadelphia, and they married in 1882. In 1887 their daughter was born, and Louise Blum continued both as a mother and a physician. Reverend Blum and his family were transferred to the First Moravian Church of York, Pennsylvania, and in 1891, Louise opened a new private practice there. But she retired from active medical practice in 1897, when Reverend Blum was elected principal of Nazareth Hall Military Academy and invited his wife to serve with him as "lady principal." She accepted, and as her obituary described her choice, "ended her medical career in order to devote herself entirely to the school work, which in an institution of such a nature is necessarily the joint work of husband and wife."[20]

Dr. Louise Schneider Blum died in 1923, having practiced medicine for half her working life and having served beside her husband to educate the rising generation in the other half. Her obituary characterized both aspects of her career as part of one effort. In the academy, it recorded, "her splendid qualities showed themselves in the excellence of her schoolwork as they had showed themselves in her medical practice." Teaching and healing, educating and curing were taken by Blum and her generation to be equal and compatible responsibilities of women who served society.

Martha Dunn Corey

None of the Woman's Medical College classmates who graduated with Martha Dunn in 1879 might have expected that the shy young woman from upstate New York would enjoy one of the most traveled and long-lived careers among them. Martha Dunn Corey's career carried her from a quiet rural practice across the entire United States to La Jolla, California, where she became that community's first physician. In her medical trek across America, she married, raised three children, and involved herself in the local activities and medical societies of each community in which she and her family resided. Though never permanently settled until near the end of her career, Martha Dunn Corey nevertheless proved to be a remarkable successful physician. At her death in 1927, she left an estate of over eighty-two thousand dollars.

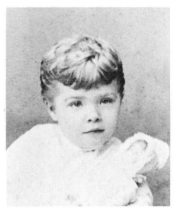

Edith Blum, daughter of Dr. Louise Schneider Blum and Reverend Samuel J. Blum (1890s). Petrulias Family Collection.

Martha Dunn Corey was born August 18, 1852, in New York City. Orphaned when she was still young, she was adopted by the Reverend and Mrs. H. M. Danforth and raised by them in Evans, New York. There Martha attended public school and private academies, and for a time, worked as a teacher. In 1876 she graduated from the Woman's Homeopathic College of New York and the following year enrolled in the Woman's Medical College of Pennsylvania. She graduated with the Class of 1879, at age twenty-seven.

Martha Dunn Corey then began a career that would take her to at least six communities in a practice that spanned forty-four years. She began in Utica, New York, in private practice with former classmate Dr. Charlotte Merrick, with whom she worked through 1882. In 1883 she moved to Waterbury, Connecticut, where she practiced for the next five years. In the summer of 1887 she took leave to study surgery in Birmingham, England, with the renowned surgeon Dr. Lawson Tait. Returning home at summer's end, she met George Henry Corey aboard ship. They courted and were married the following spring.

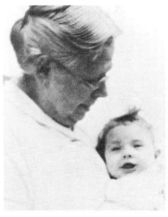

Dr. Louise Schneider Blum with granddaughter, Louise Petrulias (1921). Petrulias Family Collection.

The Coreys' marriage proved to be a stormy one, strained by continued years of changing communities and practices. They began their married life in Springfield, Missouri, about 1889, where they seemed to have remained through 1891. By mid-1891 they were living in Circleville, Ohio, near the West Virginia border, and in late 1891, their first son was born. In 1892, by train and stagecoach, Martha moved her small family across the country to Pacific Beach, California, near La Jolla. There, in her home, she established a general and obstetrical practice, becoming the region's first resident physician.

In 1893, a second son was born to the Coreys, and Martha's practice continued to grow. They remained in the Pacific Beach/La Jolla area until 1900,

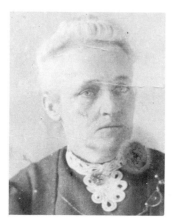

Dr. Martha Dunn Corey.
Corey Family Collection.

when the family moved back to Marion, Ohio. There, where the Coreys remained for the next six years, her third and last son was born. Conflicting records about divorce proceedings and abandonment indicate the Coreys' marriage was seriously troubled, but by 1906 Martha was widowed, and she returned to what she seems to have considered her only true home, La Jolla.

For the next seventeen years, Martha conducted her private practice in La Jolla, raising her family and involving herself in community and civic affairs. As the summer communities and general population of Southern California grew, so too did her practice. She retired from medicine in 1923, and when she died in 1927, at age seventy-five she left an estate of $82,610.47.

Dr. Martha Dunn Corey's will crystalized the astonishing success of La Jolla's first physicians. She left twenty-five thousand dollars to her stepbrother, and another one thousand dollars to the Woman's Medical College of Pennsylvania. The remainder of her estate was set in trust for her two surviving sons. (Her youngest son, a physician, had predeceased her.) In addition, her son William inherited her oriental rug, her radio, and a portrait of her father. To her son Frederick, she left "my Ford automobile,"[21] an "air-cooled Franklin [in which] she had her sons drive her up and down La Jolla Boulevard with flags flying, bells ringing, and chickens running."[22] Her career had taken her from upstate New York to the boomtowns of Southern California; from the horse-and-buggy age to the age of the automobile. Along the way she had survived a bad marriage, raised three children, amassed a sizeable estate, and earned herself a place in the memory of her community. Having outlived most of her medical school classmates, she had thrived in a world few of them could have imagined. But she had navigated that world, and succeeded in it, with the skills nurtured in her by the nineteenth century.

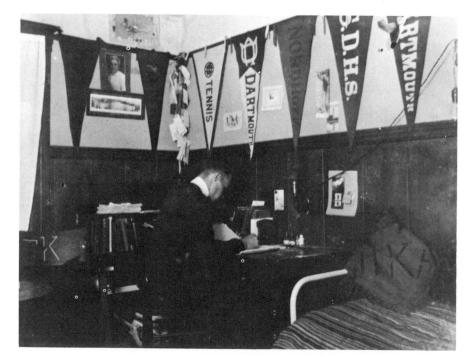

The Dartmouth College dormitory room of Dr. Martha Dunn Corey's son (c. 1910). His mother's picture hangs below nude on wall. Corey Family Collection.

Mary Wolfenden Battershall

Mary Wolfenden Battershall's signalled a life and career that nearly exemplified the best expectations for nineteenth-century women physicians. She was born on September 18, 1854, in New York City, the middle child of five siblings. By the time she was a schoolgirl, her family had settled in Attleboro, Massachusetts, where Mary attended the public schools and began to teach after her graduation. In 1876, she enrolled in the Woman's Medical College of Pennsylvania, graduating three years later.

Wolfenden Battershall's early postgraduate career followed the established pattern for many of her contemporaries. In 1881 she joined the staff of the New England Hospital for Women and Children, extending her training under women physicians and specializing in related medical practice. The following year she went to work in the Nursery and Child's Hospital on Staten Island. By the mid-80s, she had returned to her hometown of Attleboro where, in 1887, she married the physician and surgeon Dr. Joseph Battershall. In their home at 12 Park Street, they established a successful joint private practice, and the Attleboro directories for those years list "Battershall, Joseph W., physician and surgeon" above a line that reads, "Battershall, Mary W. Mrs., physician."[23] They attracted a "large clientele of patients" and "were known most widely . . . for the interest and attention they displayed."[24]

Dr. Mary Wolfenden Battershall's interests also drew her into lively professional and community activity. A member of the Massachusetts Medical Society from 1911 until her death in 1928, she was, as well, a lifelong member of the Attleboro Doctor's Club. She worked actively throughout her career for woman's suffrage and served on local and state Republican committees. She seems to have achieved a certain political as well as medical prominence, working for better health programs and living standards for her community.

In 1893, at age thirty-nine, she gave birth to the Battershalls' only son, Jesse, who in his turn became a physician, graduating from Tufts Medical School with honors in 1916. Jesse Battershall, too, returned to Attleboro, where he eventually became a school physician and the district medical examiner. When he died unexpectedly in May 1945, his obituary in the Attleboro paper credited the son's career in medicine—and its orientation to community service—to the influence of his parents and the breed of nineteenth-century medicine to which they subscribed:

> It is natural that Dr. [Jesse] Battershall had absorbed from his parents the ideal that healing and comfort of the sick, in all walks of life, and promotion of better health and living conditions for all was a foremost work in the household. . . . Dr. Battershall stepped into an atmosphere in which service to the community, with old-fashioned ideals of humanity and self-sacrifice, was long a watchword.[25]

NOTES

1. Phoebe Flagler (Hagenbuch) and Agnes Kemp were married before they entered the Woman's Medical College of Pennsylvania. Flagler's husband died during the second year of her studies. Agnes Kemp had been widowed twice by the time she

entered medical school, at the age of fifty-two. Mina Fitch Wood was married before she entered the college, at age twenty-three, although no records mention a husband after her graduation in 1879.

2. Regina Markell Morantz, "The 'Connecting Link': The Case for the Woman Doctor in Nineteenth-Century America," in *Sickness and Health in America: Readings in the History of Medicine and Public Health*, Judith Walzer Leavitt and Ronald Numbers, eds. (Madison: University of Wisconsin Press, 1978), *passim.*

3. Lucy Weaver Soule, "Women in Medicine: A Ministering Angel at Whose Touch Every Door Should Open," speech before the Rhode Island Women's Club, February 20, 1884; Archives and Special Collections on Women in Medicine, Medical College of Pennsylvania.

4. According to Regina Morantz-Sanchez, between one-fifth and one-third of women doctors overall in the late nineteenth century married. See her "From Art to Science: Women Physicians in American Medicine, 1600–1980," in *In Her Own Words: Oral Histories of Women Physicians* (Westport, CT: Greenwood Press, 1982), __. See also Mary Roth Walsh, *"Doctors Wanted: No Women Need Apply": Sexual Barriers in the Medical Profession, 1835–1975* (New Haven, CT: Yale University Press, 1977), 184, following an 1881 survey of practicing American women physicians by doctors Emily F. Pope, Emma L. Call, and C. Augusta Pope, which suggests 41 percent of women physicians married.

5. If Phoebe Flagler (who remarried after graduation at age thirty-six) is removed from the list, the average age of marriage is twenty-nine.

6. Board of Public Charities of Pennsylvania, *Third Report of the Commission on Lunacy,* September 30, 1985.

7. Portland (Maine) *Post*, October 11, 1904.

8. Portland *Post*.

9. Morantz-Sanchez, "From Art to Science," 8.

10. Nellie Blessing Eyster, *A Noted Mother and Daughter* (San Francisco: Tomoye Press, 190), 2; Lawrence Family Collection.

11. Ibid., 2.

12. Ibid., 4.

13. Ibid., 14.

14. Ibid., 12.

15. Ibid., 14.

16. Ibid., 15.

17. Ibid., 42.

18. Ibid.

19. Bethelehem (Pennsylvania) *Globe-Times,* October 13, 1923.

20. Bethlehem *Globe-Times*.

21. Last Will and Testament of Martha Dunn Corey, January 20, 1927, San Diego, California. Archives and Special Collections on Women and Medicine, Medical College of Pennsylvania; Corey Family Collection.

22. *The Bulletin of the San Diego Medical Society,* October, 1971, Archives and Special Collections on Women in Medicine, Medical College of Pennsylvania; Corey Family Collection.

23. See, for example, the Attleboro (Massachusetts) City Directory for 1905.

24. Attleboro (Massachusetts) *Sun,* May 4, 1928.

25. Attleboro *Sun,* May 1945.

Part Four

RELAPSE/DIAGNOSIS

The Turn-of-the-Century Decline of Women Physicians

Never have women . . . been so respected, so honored, so . . . loved as they are right now.

—Dr. Elizabeth Carpenter, 1919

Introduction

APPEARING in 1919 before the sixty-seventh graduating class of the Woman's Medical college of Pennsylvania, Dr. Elizabeth Carpenter argued in behalf of separate medical schools for women and made optimistic predictions for the future of women physicians, indeed, for all women. "Never," said Carpenter, "have women . . . been so respected, so honored, so . . . loved as they are right now."[1] Yet even as she spoke, medical women were in trouble, as the following essay by Regina Morantz-Sanchez so clearly explains. The reasons are many and complex and the subject of serious debate among scholars. It is hoped that by understanding the forces that contributed to the setback, light may be shed on the question of how any group outside the dominant culture can sustain hard-won social, political, and economic gains.

Dr. Carpenter assured the new graduates that "never was there a greater need for doctors."[2] Yet, as she well knew, the existence of a great need for doctors would not ensure women a secure place in the medical profession. Ironically, it was Dr. Carpenter herself who told the story of how the American officers refused to allow women physicians to serve in World War I at the very moment when they "faced the last dreadful drive from the enemy, and when there was a dire need of immediate aid and skillful relief for the wounded and suffering men. . . ."[3] Rebuffed, the American volunteers went to the French, who accepted them and awarded their meritorious service under fire with the Croix de Guerre.

In a twist of fate, the women's medical movement slid backward just when it seemed victory was at hand. The opening of some of America's most

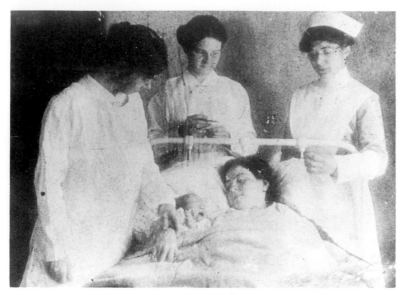

Dr. Alice Weld Talent, Dr. Helen Taylor (intern), and nurse with patient in the maternity ward, Hospital of the Woman's Medical College of Pennsylvania (1915). ASCWM, MCP.

prestigious medical schools to women obscured some of the more subtle changes that would serve to diminish the number of women physicians.

Morantz-Sanchez discusses the impact of the change in the view of women that transpired beginning in the late nineteenth century. Other observers have offered additional arguments. Mary Roth Walsh suggests that "the declining sexual taboos [shrunk] what had once been a guaranteed market for women physicians"[4] among Victorian women too modest to seek medical help from a male physician.

To support her contention that women were well loved, Dr. Carpenter cited the establishment of Mother's Day as a national holiday. Indeed, there was a new focus on mothers and with it a new pressure on women to stay home. Findings in the new field of psychiatry suggested, according to Barbara Ehrenreich and Deirdre English, that the child was no longer " 'a mere incident in the preservation of the species' but the potential link to a higher plateau of evolutionary development. It fell to the mother to forge that link. Motherhood could no longer be seen as a biological condition or a part-time occupation; it was becoming a noble calling."[5] Dr. Eliza Taylor Ransom, a Boston physician noted for her pioneering work in the "twilight sleep" method of childbirth, was one of many who coached women back into the home. In an article published in 1927, Dr. Ransom told the story of a "mannish" woman, now in her forties, who had bought wholesale that "hateful slogan of the earlier suffragists" and had heeded her mother's counsel to "do something for yourself." Spurning marriage, the woman built a successful legal career, only to regret it. "My life," she told Ransom, "is a terrible waste. A tragedy. A failure. Today, I want marriage, a man to love me, a home where I am queen. I'd give ten years of my life if I could have a child of my own."[6]

The decline of the women's movement also affected the women's medical movement. "Twenty years after . . . suffrage," William Chafe explained, "the women's rights movement had reached a nadir. It had ceased to exist as a powerful force in American society."[7] It was a movement to which nineteenth-century women doctors had been deeply committed. Walsh points out that of the women physicians included in *Notable American Women,* 96 percent either were affiliated with women's institutions or were leaders in the nineteenth-century women's movement.[8]

Estelle Friedman has suggested that the "erosion of women's culture," a hallmark of the Victorian era, may "account for the decline of public feminism after 1920. . . . The old feminist leaders lost their following when a new generation opted for assimilation in the hope of becoming men's equals overnight."[9] By 1900, Dr. Mary Putnam Jacobi, who was one of those leaders, identified woman's lack of class interest as a major problem.[10]

Viewing themselves as social housekeepers, nineteenth-century women physicians had also played a role in the health and hygiene movement. They applauded the passage of the Shepard-Towner Act, which made children's health and women's prenatal care and education an explicit function of the state. Women physicians were to be hired to fulfill the act's mandate. However, this avenue for continued service was blocked just a year later when the American Medical Association lobbied successfully against the act.[11]

As Morantz-Sanchez suggests, changes in the location of medical care also had an impact on women physicians. No longer could they promise, as had Dr. Ann Preston, that the pursuit of a medical career would not cause them to abandon the "holy hearth of home."[12] More important, the relocation of medical care from the home to the hospital removed the home-based office, with its attendant convenience for a physician balancing home and family, to the periphery of medical care. Nineteenth-century feminist thinker Charlotte Perkins Gilman argued that "unless the home itself as well as its relation to the workplace was constituted in some fundamental fashion, unification of the separate spheres of women's lives would not be possible."[13]

Even the change nineteenth-century women physicians had fought hardest for—coeducation—had its drawbacks. When Dr. Emily Blackwell announced the closing of the Woman's Medical College of Pennsylvania, she noted with regret that the decision ended the careers of many fine female professors. It was understood that while Cornell and Johns Hopkins and other medical

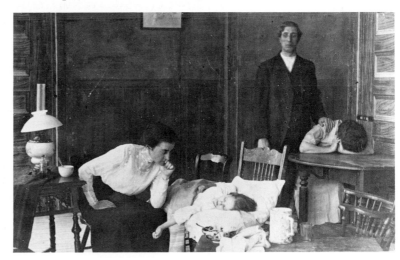

Dr. Agnes Hockaday on house call (c. 1920).
ASCWM, MCP.

schools accepted women students, they had no intention of adding women to their faculties. Speaking in 1912, Dr. Alice Weld Talent, who had received her medical degree at a coeducational school, explained that without a female role model, a woman was bound to think that she could not do the task as well as a man, "no matter how strongly you feel in favor of women."[14]

The escalating cost of the newly scientific medical education created a problem for women. Nineteenth-century female medical students tended to come from families that were struggling to maintain middle-class status. Members of the class of 1879 discussed earlier, came from families with more than the average number of children to support. This, the fathers' occupations, and in many cases their deaths often left the families in strained circumstances. As long as a woman earning a teacher's salary could garner sufficient monies to support a medical education, she had a chance. But when tuitions were raised, those chances were dimmed. There had never been a tradition of well-to-do women electing a medical career.

Dr. Carpenter ended her address by urging the class to move "forward," assuring them they need not fear even a "mole hill of dread."[15] Neither she nor the graduates could yet perceive the roadblocks in their paths.

NOTES

1. Elizabeth Carpenter, M.D., Address, Annual Commencement of the Woman's Medical College of Pennsylvania, 1919.
2. Ibid.
3. Ibid.
4. Mary Roth Walsh, "*Doctors Wanted: No Women Need Apply*": Sexual Barriers in the Medical Profession, 1835–1975 (New Haven, CT: Yale University Press, 1977), 261.
5. Barbara Ehrenreich and Deirdre English, *For Her Own Good: 150 Years of the Experts' Advice to Women,* (New York: Anchor Press/Doubleday, 1979), 189.
6. Eliza Ransom, M.D., "Shall We Teach Them," August 1927. Magazine, untitled, in Schlesinger Library, Radcliffe College.
7. William Chafe, *The American Woman: Her Changing Social, Economic and Political Role, 1920–1970,* (London: Oxford Press, 1972), 132.
8. Walsh, "*Doctors Wanted,*" 261.
9. Estelle Friedman, "Separatism as Strategy: Female Institution Building and American Feminism, 1870–1930," *Feminist Studies* 5, no. 3 (Fall 1979): 515.
10. Walsh, "*Doctors Wanted,*" 265.
11. William Leach, *True Love and Perfect Union, The Feminist Reform of Sex and Society* (New York: Basic Books, 1980), 350.
12. Dr. Ann Preston, M.D., Address, Annual Commencement of the Woman's Medical College of Pennsylvania.
13. Joyce Antler, "Feminism as Life-Process: The Life and Career of Lucy Sprague Mitchell," *Feminist Studies* 7, no. 7 (Spring 1984): 146.
14. Alice Weld Talent, M.D., Address, Annual Commencement of the Woman's Medical College of Pennsylvania, 1912.
15. Elizabeth Carpenter, M.D., Address, Annual Commencement of the Woman's Medical College of Pennsylvania, 1919.

So Honored, So Loved?

The Women's Medical Movement in Decline

REGINA MORANTZ-SANCHEZ

L IKE other social feminists at the end of the nineteenth century, women physicians boasted a measure of achievement that offered ample opportunity for pride and satisfaction. In numbers alone they had increased by several thousand and in 1900 comprised close to 5 percent of the profession.[1] Visionary women like Elizabeth Blackwell, Mary Putnam Jacobi, Ann Preston, Marie Zakrzewska, and Mary Harris Thompson could point proudly to the medical schools and hospitals that educated and trained first-rate women physicians in several major cities. Perhaps even more promising from their perspective was the progress on medical coeducation. A number of midwestern universities had begun to acccept women students. By 1900, for example, the University of Michigan had trained 394 women in its medical department.[2] The crowning achievement in this field was the opening of Johns Hopkins University Medical School in 1893. Through the combined efforts of Bryn Mawr dean M. Carey Thomas, prominent female medical educators, and a network of committed feminists, the school agreed to admit women on the same terms as men. In return, Thomas and her friends gave the institution a total of $500,000 in contributions. Without this money, the medical school never would have become a reality. Thomas and her contemporaries rightly believed this achievement to be a crucial event in the history of American feminism.[3]

231

Other developments, too, provided cause for optimism. With the decline of sectarian medicine, 75 percent or more of women doctors were regular physicians. This development gave them as a group more credibility within the profession, which was moving rapidly toward standardization and orthodoxy. During the last third of the nineteenth century, most state and local medical societies quietly admitted women without objection.[4] Although the American Medical Association did not formally accept women until 1915, it indirectly recognized them when it received Dr. Sarah Hackett Stevenson as a state delegate from Illinois at the 1876 convention. Women physicians had also made progress in gaining admission to hospital clerkships, especially in New York, Philadelphia, and Chicago. Motivated either by custom or by law, several states had begun to appoint women physicians as clinicians or superintendents at state asylums in which women were confined.[5] In addition, a handful of women surgeons had managed to demonstrate proficiency in a specialty that was gaining visible status within the profession. Other women doctors could look with pride at the growing list of publications by women in respected scientific and medical journals.[6]

Furthermore, women physicians had taken steps to formalize professional networks among themselves. In the decade between 1890 and 1900, women's medical societies were founded in many states.[7] Those in Boston and New York were particularly strong. In Philadelphia, the alumnae association of the Woman's Medical College of Pennsylvania was especially active; in 1900 it boasted 219 members. Because it had a policy of giving honorary membership to distinguished female graduates of other schools, this association, which met for several days annually, offered much more than mere parochial social contact. Members read and criticized each other's scientific papers, which were then published in the alumnae journal. They also shared case studies, debated such professional issues as fee splitting and specialization, and took positive steps to promote the interests of women in the profession. In 1893, a group of women physicians from Toledo, Ohio, began the *Woman's Medical Journal,* a periodical devoted to raising professional consciousness by publishing both scientific articles and material about women physicians culminated in 1915 with the founding of the American Medical Women's Association by a group of Chicago women.[8]

As the new century wore on, however, decisive changes within the organization of the medical profession and profound shifts in cultural beliefs regarding a woman's role and activity in the public and private spheres called the achievements of nineteenth-century medical women into question. More than one historian has portrayed the years between 1900 and 1965 as dark ones for the progress of women in medicine, as years in which nineteenth-century beachheads were surrendered and lost to male backlash and institutional discrimination.[9]

A glance at the statistics appears to confirm such a view. Despite the enormous promise of coeducation in the 1890s, the ranks of women physicians did not continue to increase. In fact, the number of women medical students actually declined from 1,280 to 992 in the years between 1902 and 1926. Female physicians lost ground both in percentages and in absolute numbers. Moreover, the charts reveal that medicine was the only profession in which the numbers of women declined absolutely. After peaking at 6 percent of the national total in 1910, the percentages steadily shrank, and only in 1950 did women physicians again reach the magic 6 percent. It was not until the 1970s that dramatic alterations in the numbers of women in medical schools again occurred.[10]

Although the reasons for the declining numbers of medical women in the first half of the twentieth century are complicated, one significant factor, often slighted by historians, is the enormous alteration that came about in the structure and content of the medical care delivery system.

It is important to remember that the modern medical profession grew to maturity in the first three decades of the twentieth century. At the beginning of this period, issues of professionalization took center stage, as the roles of professional associations, state licensing agencies, and colleges and universities only gradually emerged into their modern forms. In 1900, the majority of physicians believed that their economic and social position, as well as the collective status of the profession itself, warned of a crisis in medicine. Probably for the first time, the interests of various competing groups within the profession—medical societies, eastern scientific elites, midwestern general practitioners, licensing agencies, and the leading bloc of medical colleges—pointed to the necessity for consolidation and reform. Common aims included the raising of professional entrance standards, the standardization of medical school curricula, the suppression of weak proprietary institutions, and the overall reduction in the number of medical graduates. The educational goal of raising standards remained decisively intertwined with the policy of drastically reducing the number of practitioners in a field believed already to be overcrowded.[11]

By critically analyzing the medical reform movement, recent historical scholarship has contributed much toward an understanding of medicine as an instrument of social control. A few social historians also have demonstrated the medical profession's central role in promoting its own interests in these years. Doctors clearly intended to upgrade their status and income as well as their professional skills. Finally, researchers tentatively have begun to clarify what they see as a link between reform strategies and a more general ideological support for the dominant industrial classes and the specific interests of a capitalistic corporate state.[12] Viewing the medical reform movement from the perspective of this recent work provides a clearer understanding of the effect of modern medical professionalism on women.

Perhaps the most immediate problem facing the reformers was the large number of inferior schools. Working through the joint efforts of the American Medical Association Council on Medical Education, the publicity and the public pressure provided by the *Journal of the American Medical Association,* and the offices of several state licensing boards, the leaders of medical reform began the process of self-criticism. Yet pressure from within was perhaps even less significant in the long run than pressure from without. It was in this period that large philanthropic foundations backed by the Rockefeller and Carnegie wealth began to use their resources to force specific changes in medical education and research. From 1910 to 1930 foundations donated over $300 million to medical education and research. Indeed, Rosemary Stevens

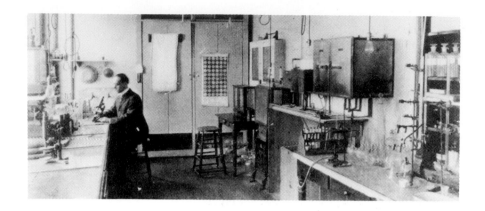

Pathological-Chemical Laboratory (1909). Central Dispensary and Emergency Hospital.

has argued that these philanthropic foundations were "the most vital outside source in effecting changes in medical education after 1910."[13]

The most crucial historical event in this new alliance between scientific medicine and corporate power was the Carnegie Foundation's publication in 1910 of Abraham Flexner's meticulous study of contemporary medical education. The Flexner report made public what medical educators had known privately and had worked to correct for a decade: American medical schools labored under appalling inadequacies. Most schools accepted inferior students, provided meager or nonexistent training in laboratory science and clinical medicine, and overproduced doctors. Only the youthful Johns Hopkins University Medical School totally escaped Flexner's scathing criticism. According to Flexner's study, medical schools needed to be placed under the control of universities; preliminary education requirements needed to be placed under the control of universities; preliminary education requirements needed to be enforced; curricula needed to be lengthened; and laboratory facilities needed to be improved. These changes would please both the foundations, which wanted higher standards, and the profession, which wanted less competition.

And there was more. The need to decrease the number of doctors and consolidate medical schools reflected one important aspect of medical reform; the affiliation of surviving schools with hospitals and dispensaries reflected yet another. The hospital already had begun gradually to concentrate the complex technology that became the hallmark of modern medicine within its walls. Indeed, the leading spokesmen for scientific medicine regarded the hospital as so essential to the medical school curriculum that, in 1900, the *Journal of the American Medical Association* declared, "to a large extent, the hospital, with [all its facilities] *is* the medical school."[14]

Flexner remained adamant on all his recommedations, and although his candid study did not launch the process of medical reform, which was already underway, it probably hastened the results. Between 1904 and 1915, 92 schools merged or closed their doors when confronted with higher state board requirements, poor clinical facilities, financial difficulties, or Flexner's public criticism. By 1920, only 85 out of the 155 medical schools visited by Flexner remained in existence.[15] The better schools improved their facilities through the generous help of the foundations; others were left to fend for themselves. Unfortunately, but not surprisingly, among those schools denied the largesse of the new philanthropy were the three women's medical schools that had survived into the twentieth century.[16]

The reasons for the failure of all but one of the women's medical schools to survive past the second decade of the twentieth century are complex and cannot be explained merely be raising the ugly specter of discrimination. Discrimination certainly did exist, but it is also true that medical women were hampered by the limitations of and contradictions in their own ideology, an ideology no longer suited to the problems of the new century.[17]

In a very real sense, the goals of the nineteenth-century women's medical movement had been realized by the opening decade of the new century. Women physicians had fought for equal opportunities in medical education on philosophical grounds that unquestionably accepted women's dominance over the private sphere. Indeed, they never had anticipated women's participation in medicine to be on the same level as men's, nor had they expected or desired that the majority of women would leave home for full-time, extradomestic activity. They understood that the woman physician would always remain exceptional. In fact, they fought unabashedly for the rights of that exceptional minority. They fully believed that the realization of those rights would benefit society at large because women physicians naturally were better than men in treating women and children, concerned themselves more assiduously with preventative medicine, and worked in a more general sense to humanize the profession by weaning it away from narrow self-interest. It was only in the altered cultural setting of the twentieth century that nineteenth-century goals began to shift to a more broadly egalitarian position.

To be sure, women physicians never demonstrated a thorough unanimity when they mustered their arguments in defense of woman's medical education. Although there was a strong tendency to emphasize their unique contributions, a few hardheaded scientists, like Mary Putnam Jacobi, coolly deplored such sentimentalism. Although Jacobi never entirely discarded the notion that women had special strengths, she feared that such an ideology led to female-centered, moralistic, separatist standards. In contrast to these, her assumptions remained fundamentally universalistic and assimilationist.[18] Jacobi's approach, however, proved distinctly less popular in the public and private thought of women doctors until the twentieth century. And, as we shall see, assimilation exacted its own price.

Ironically, despite an ideology that emphasized their own uniqueness, few women physicians favored separate education or understood the potential pitfalls of medical coeducation. With the exception of the faculty of the Woman's Medical College of Pennsylvania, female medical educators looked at the women's schools as temporary expedients. In fact, women physicians seem to have been haunted periodically by the fear that women could not maintain first-rate educational facilities by themselves. By the close of the nineteenth century, burdened with the rising financial costs of quality medical education and heartened by the prospects for equal opportunity at existing male schools, female institutions passed out of existence one by one. It could be argued that in so doing, female medical educators lost, however unwittingly, the autonomous control of institutions that, at least in the case of Chicago and New York, had provided an opportunity for a self-supporting and self-directed female community to inspire younger women to follow in its footsteps. Coeducation never fulfilled its promise, and women physicians continued to find themselves isolated as a group from the mainstream of American medicine.[19]

During this period of assimilation, the Woman's Medical College of Pennsylvania limped along, a sole dissenter in the ranks. Skeptical of the rewards of coeducation for all types of women, its faculty struggled valiantly in the face of staggering financial difficulties to maintain a class A rating with the American Medical Association. One cannot help wondering what feats this school could have accomplished had it received the $500,000 endowment M. Carey Thomas and Mary Elizabeth Garrett gave to John Hopkins. Instead, the Woman's Medical College of Pennsylvania fell victim to women physicians' collective attitude toward separate education. Over the years, more and more men took important positions on its faculty, which helped the school maintain an aura of legitimacy in the harsh professional realities of the modern medical world. While praising the college for its "striking evidence of a genuine effort to do the best possible with limited resources," Abraham Flexner then went on to reiterate the arguments of Dean Emily Blackwell when she announced in 1899 the merger of the New York Infirmary with Cornell University. Flexner observed:

> Medical education is now, in the United States and Canada, open to women upon practically the same terms as men. If all institutions do not receive women, so many do, that no woman desiring an education in medicine is under any disability in finding a school to which she may gain admittance. . . . Woman has so apparent a function in certain medical specialities and seemingly so assured a place in general medicine under some obvious limitations that the struggle for wider educational opportunities for the sex was predestined to an early success. . . . Whether it is either wise or necessary to endow separate medical schools for women is a problem. . . . In the first place, eighty percent of women who have in the last six years studied medicine have attended coeducational institutions. None of the three women's medical colleges now existing can be sufficiently strengthened without enormous outlay. . . . In the general need of more liberal support for medical schools, it would appear that large sums, as far as specially available for the medical education of women, would accomplish most if used to develop coeducational institutions in which their benefits would be shared by men without loss to women students.[20]

Tension between separatism and assimilation has continued to divide women physicians, as it has other minority groups, in the twentieth century. With the achievement of coeducation, militant separatism understandably appeared to many to threaten the posibility that men would welcome women colleagues as equals. It seemed to the younger women physicians that the battle over equal intelligence had ended, and they lacked the pioneer determination of their elders because significant advances in fact had been made. Consequently, many women rejected formal contacts with professional women's associations. Others unwittingly internalized cultural assumptions that were suspicious of separatist institutions and groups. As a result, only the most militant and feminist women joined the American Medical Women's Association after 1915. Although the organization has not only advanced the cause of women in medicine but also supported such various sociomedical issues as liberalized birth control laws, medical insurance, Medicaid, Medicare, and abortion reform, its membership rolls have never attracted more than one-third of the women physicians in the country.[21]

The younger generations of women physicians, for whom sex discrimination was often so subtle that it went unnoticed, were uncomfortable with the feminist militancy of the American Medical Women's Association. Many shared the sentiments of Ethel Walker, a pediatric resident at Johns Hopkins Hospital, who in 1940 explained to Bertha Van Hoosen, a prominent surgeon and the founder of the American Medical Women's Association, her reasons for not joining the organization:

> I am strongly opposed to any organization or individual's attitude which sets women apart from men . . . instead of teaching them to lose themselves in their profession. . . . In the early days of women in medicine they no doubt had to band together, but now in most sections of the country if not all, the quicker the woman physician can forget any feeling that she is in a class apart from her men colleagues the happier she will be and the better she and they will get along. In medical school and interne days I have seen it happen time and time again that the girls who were totally unconscious of any difference between themselves and their men confreres and who mingled with them on exactly the same footing achieved a professional equality and friendship which was entirely denied to the women who were always huddled together with other women and who continually made it plain to everybody that they were different and knew they were different. In my experience it has been the former group who did well in their profession . . . whereas other group of women's women . . . seldom advanced.[22]

The late-nineteenth-century scientific revolution in medical therapeutics also produced tension within the ranks of women physicians and disarmed the arguments that earlier women physicians had used in support of female medical education. Nineteenth-century suppositions about the body had described illness as a phenomenon of the total organism. Physicians who wished to restore a patient's health did so by readjusting the body's internal equilibrium and returning it to harmony with its enviroment. Under these assumptions, local inflammations were indicative of systemic ills, and localized treatment was intended to remedy general physical states. Before taking action, the experienced physician weighed a bewildering complexity of factors that included climate, age, gender, and the family's constitutional idiosyncrasies. The better he knew the patient, the better his chances for success, for each individual organism displayed its own distinct features and interacted uniquely with a constantly changing environment.[23]

In contrast to this, the major theme pervading the history of modern therapeutics is that of discreteness and specificity. When bacteriologists directed their attention to specific symptoms and causes, they revolutionized the approach to disease. No longer is medication selected to effect a balance in the entire organism. Therapy is aimed at discrete entities, and the intention is to remove the causes altogether. In this view of disease, somatic considerations reign supreme, and there is little room for the social, psychological and behavioral dimensions of illness. As a consequence, both the physician's approach to his own discipline and the public's perception of his role have changed considerably.

Whereas the nineteenth-century physician approached his patient with a predisposition to physiological holism, twentieth-century therapeutics have transformed the doctor into a specialist whose knowledge encompasses some specific symptom or some discrete portion of the patient's body. Treatment understandably has become fragmented; total patient "care" has become increasingly dissociated from the specialist's concerns as he busies himself with patient "cure." Indeed, medicine has become so identified with this highly technical and reductionist approach that for many physicians whatever lies outside the domain of specific diagnosis and treatment lies outside the domain of medicine itself.[24]

Institutional developments in the early twentieth century reflected this gradual fragmentation in the delivery of health care. The general practitioner became an endangered species. Physicians even became alienated gradually from one another as each specialty developed its own language and body of knowledge. As doctors found it less necessary to treat patients in their homes, care shifted to the hospital, which offered a more convenient setting for the highly technical and narrower approach to disease.[25] Gradually, nurses and social workers took on the nineteenth-century physician's heuristic role. Public health nurses, for example, replaced the women interns who had defiantly entered the slums to teach the poor how to be well. In their effort to professionalize and claim nursing for women, self-conscious leaders in the field of nursing played an important part in shifting the so-called feminine and nurturant aspects of medical care from the doctor to the nurse. In 1913, while struggling to define an independent role for the tuberculosis nurse, Elizabeth Gregg, superintendent of nurses for the New York City Health Department, wrote:

> Physicians have not the time, neither is it born in many [doctors] to devote themselves to the detail that requires the patient, painstaking effort of a woman; and this detail tends to reveal the very causes or the contributing factors of tuberculosis more than in any other disease; so that the nurse, with her knowledge of home conditions and the family's principles of living, and with her instinctive woman's insight into the causes of trouble, is the physician's right hand.[26]

Although women doctors were not alone in their sensitivity to such changes in the field, they often lamented the passing of the "human" in the practice of medicine. Eliza Mosher, for example, a past president of the American Medical Women's Association, regretted the loss of "the sympathetic relation which formerly existed between doctors and their patients," and warned her colleagues to beware of "narrowing and concentrating their vision upon the purely physical to the exclusion of the psychic and human."[27] Others continued to believe that medical women were obliged to exert their influence in favor of more holistic approaches. In 1930, M. Esther Harding, a psychiatrist, spoke for many women doctors when she wrote to Bertha Van Hoosen,

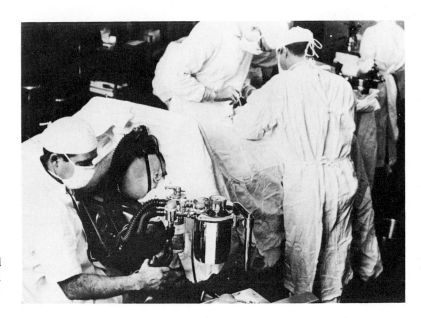

Surgeons in operating room (1960). Medical archives, New York Hospital/Cornell Medical Center.

I have been struck recently more than once at the meetings of a Psychotherapeutic Society of which I am a member with a queer little difference between the attitude and approach [*sic*] of the men and the women . . . to the subject under discussion. . . . Usually the men lead off with scientifically arranged data, followed by statistics and rather abstract theory. Then presently a woman speaks up and nearly always her voice is raised to remind the group that after all the patient is a human being and not merely the subject of certain symptoms or mechanisms. And this I think is characteristic. We women are more nearly concerned with the human problem presented to us and relatively less absorbed with the collection and classification of scientific material. Let us who write about the intricacies of the human psyche, whether in its normal functioning or in its illnesses and conflicts, remember always that in any final analysis it is the human being that matters. Knowledge of disease and its detailed investigation are not ends in themselves, they are only means to an end, namely that the human being may grow and flourish.[28]

Even in the fragmented and technocratic context of the early twentieth century, women continued to preserve their penchant for holistic approaches through their specialty choices, which usually fell into the primary care fields, most notably general practice, pediatrics, and psychiatry.[29] Public-health work, especially part-time positions with low pay and little prestige, also attracted a steady stream of women. It simply cannot be argued convincingly that their involvement in public-health work was caused only by their "exclusion from other medical careers due to sex discrimination."[30] Women doctors seemed to be well suited for public-health work, and no one argued this point more forcefully than they themselves. Married women physicians, who needed more flexible time commitments in order to care for their families, were urged by leading women in the field to choose school and community work. The history of the anonymous women physicians who filled important social needs as clinical workers for the Federal Children's Bureau, part-time members of local boards of health, school physicians, and charity workers still needs to be written.[31]

Of course, the achievements of such prominent pioneers in the field as Josephine Baker, Alice Hamilton, and Ellen C. Potter inspired others, but probably the most convincing illustration of the sustaining attraction of public-health work after 1900 is found in the life of Florence Sabin. Sabin, an early graduate of Johns Hopkins University Medical School, was a protégée of the great anatomist Franklin P. Mall. Her brilliant research in anatomy and histology led to her appointment, after fifteen years on the Johns Hopkins faculty, as the first woman member of the prestigious Rockefeller Institute. After her retirement from research in 1938, she became, at the age of seventy-three, chairwoman of the governor's subcommittee on public health in her native state of Colorado and began a dramatically successful crusade for basic health reforms.[32]

Nevertheless, although many women physicians continued to regard health education as a female responsibility, technical and professional developments made medicine a very different field of endeavor than it had been only fifty years earlier. As long as medical practice remained more a matter of "art" than "science," women found themselves drawn to the work and armed with compelling reasons for claiming it as their own. Furthermore, because nineteenth-century problems of professionalization centered on the semiprivate realm of licensing, legitimacy, and the decline of heroic medicine, women who attained a medical degree could still gain an official foothold as physicians. In contrast, the organization and practice of medicine after 1900 moved from the semiprivate to the public and political realm. These circumstances may have made it more difficult for women to carve a place for themselves. What is equally apparent, however, is that women then found it less desirable to study medicine for a complicated set of reasons. This, the discriminatory donation policies of various foundations, the rapid decline of the family-based general practitioner, the fragmentation of medical care, and the transferral of medical practice from the intimate confines of the home to the impersonal setting of a hospital converged to work in various ways against the fuller participation of women as physicians in the health-care field.

Women flocked to nursing in these years. Between 1880 and 1900 the number of nurses increased from 15,601 to 120,000.[33] Another category of health workers, "physicians' and surgeons' attendants," showed an 86 percent increase in the census from 1910 to 1920. Because nursing generally attracted women from a different class background than that of women physicians, the declining number of women doctors after 1910 cannot be explained by the expansion of nursing alone. Statistics from these years would seem to indicate rather that social work and graduate school diverted some women's interests from medicine.

The years between 1890 and 1918 reveal sharp increases in the number of women doing graduate work. The percentage of female graduate students rose from 10.2 in 1890 to 41.0 in 1918. In terms of absolute numbers, this change represented a twentyfold increase, while the number of men attending graduate school increased only fivefold. After 1910, the census data suggest that many of these women were using their degrees in the new helping professions. In that year, women made up about 56 percent of the welfare workers; ten years later their absolute numbers had increased almost 200 percent. In 1910, women comprised 30 percent of the "keepers of charitable institutions"; by 1920, that percentage had increased to 38 percent. Again, the increase in actual numbers is impressive, from 2,250 in 1910 to 4,900 in 1920. Unfortunately, the census information cannot indicate what percentage of the total body of educated women were choosing welfare work and its allied fields. Nevertheless, it is possible to hypothesize that there is a distinct connection between the rising numbers of women with advanced degrees and the sharp increase in the number of women professionals in these occupations.[34]

The census data suggest that subtle cultural factors were at work. The twentieth century has witnessed unmistakable shifts in the primacy of essential Victorian values. Most notable among those changes have been the altered expectations surrounding the home, women, and family life. A prominent feature of Victorian culture was the exaltation of motherhood through the cult of domesticity. The high status afforded motherhood followed logically from the conviction that mothers were the primary agents for the transmission of cultural values. Yet despite their own glorification of motherhood, feminists had expressed a particular personal disdain for the patriarchal Victorian family. In the nineteenth century, large numbers of educated and professional women rejected marriage in favor of the pursuit of meaningful work. Opponents of higher education for women were fond of pointing out that college women married less frequently and had fewer children than did more ordinary women, and, indeed, statistics for the years between 1880 and 1920 support these claims.[35]

In the twentieth century, however, the image of woman-as-mother gradually gave way to the image of woman-as-mate. The social and economic changes in the decades before World War I created more positive attitudes toward pleasure, individual self-fulfillment, sexuality, and women's work.[36] Probably because of this altered climate, college-educated women and professional women did not continue to reject marriage with the vehemence that they had earlier. The proportion of professional women who married, for example, doubled from 12.2 percent in 1910 to 24.7 percent in 1930.[37] One historian has convincingly argued that the early twentieth century produced a new kind of feminism, previously found only among a small minority of nineteenth-century women activists. These women chose not to shun marriage but to strive instead to "work out the large issues of feminism on an individual basis." Only if we acknowledge the existence of this brand of feminism, which she labels "feminism-as-life-process," can we "rescue from the lost generation of feminist endeavor after 1920 some of the women whose lives might properly be called 'feminist.' "[38]

For those women the central issue was the need to balance participation in the public sphere through professional, political, or other activities with marriage and family. In their own lives, they struggled to "work out the balance of interestes between the private and public [in this case, between marriage and career] that would allow them to achieve the self-determination and autonomy that they posited as their highest goal." Although the number of married women physicians also increased during these years, it is quite likely that many women of this description may have been attracted to medicine initially but ruled out careers as doctors because the work appeared too strenuous, too inflexible, and ultimately less amenable to this kind of delicate balancing act.[39] It may be presumed that their choices were reinforced by the changes in medical practice itself, which was becoming increasingly more technocratic and aggressively "male."

Finally, public feminism, which had offered nineteenth-century professional women companionship and support, passed into dormancy after 1920. Older generations of women physicians occasionally mourned the passing of a "high spirit of enthusiasm for a cause" and complained of "complacency and secure smugness" among younger women doctors.[40] In fact, until the 1960s when a revitalized feminist movement used as its motto "the personal is political" and thus focused attention on the interaction between women's public and private lives, medical women engaged in intimate and solitary struggles.[41]

In explaining the decline in the number of women physicians during this period, however, the unhappy effects of institutional discrimination of all kinds must never be overlooked, even though the existence of quotas was more sporadic and decidedly less universal in medical schools than historians have believed. While schools in parts of the Northeast and South proved consistently discriminatory, others, especially in the Middle and Far West, maintained commendable percentages of female students throughout the twentieth century. From 1929 on, the percentage of acceptances for both men and women applicants hovered around 50 percent. It is apparent that the diminishing number of female students after that year paralleled the diminishing number of female applicants. When the percentage of women applicants rose in the mid-sixties so did the acceptances, although some have argued convincingly that women applicants are a more highly selective group than their male counterparts.[42]

Perhaps even more insidious than discrimination by the medical schools were the tracking systems, "old boy" networks, and women's difficulties in procuring first-rate hospital appointments. In 1914, *Harper's Weekly* complained that even female graduates from such excellent medical colleges as Cornell Medical School had problems finding good internships. Twenty years later the American Medical Women's Association revealed that almost half of the nation's hospitals had never employed a woman doctor. Although a decade later that figure had dropped to 20 percent, choice residency programs continued to remain difficult, if not impossible, to secure.[43]

In many respects, institutional discrimination was merely the most visible element of more distressing kind of exclusion. In the final analysis, women fell victim to the social dictates of a culture still characterized by extreme sex stereotyping. The vigorous, detached, almost godlike figure of the twentieth-century physician kept all but the most determined women from challenging cultural barriers. Their desire to be wives and mothers, the ambivalent feelings within the ranks of women physicians over separatism or assimilation, and the lack of an aggressive feminist movement to help them better articulate their goals made medical women an easy mark for official institutional intolerance. No one can appreciate the significance of the lives of the individual women whose stories are part of this study without understanding the complex and subtle cultural assumptions that they had to overcome.

NOTES

1. See U.S. Department of the Interior, *Report of the Commissioner of Education,* 1889–90, 1895–96,1898–99,1903 (Washington, D.C.: U.S. Government Printing Office).
2. *Alumnae Catalogue of the University of Michigan, 1837–1921* (Ann Arbor: University of Michigan Press, 1923).
3. Donald Fleming, *William H. Welch and the Rise of Modern Medicine* (Boston: Little, Brown, 1954), 96–99; M. Carey Thomas, *The Opening of the Johns Hopkins Medical School to Women,* pamphlet reprinted from *The Century Magazine* (February 1891), Sophia Smith College Collection, Northampton, MA, box labeled "Physicians U.S."; and Mary Putnam Jacobi, M.D., "Women in Medicine," in *Woman's Work in America,* ed. Annie Nathan Meyer (New York: H. Holt and Company, 1891), 205.
4. The notorious exceptions were the Massachusetts Medical Society and the Montgomery County Medical Society in Pennsylvania, both of which put up dramatic resistance, only to succumb in the 1880s. See Mary Roth Walsh, *"Doctors Wanted: No Women Need Apply," Sexual Barriers in the Medical Profession, 1835–1975* (New Haven, CT: Yale University Press, 1977), 159–65, and Jacobi, "Women in Medicine," 177–88.
5. Jacobi, "Women in Medicine," 189–96; Constance McGovern, "Predictable Failures: Women Psychiatrists and Their Patients, Pennsylvania, 1880–1910" (Paper delivered at the Organization of American Historians' Convention, San Francisco, CA, 1980).
6. Jacobi, "Woman in Medicine," 202–4; For a list of publications, see Clara Marshall, *The Woman's Medical College of Pennsylvania: an Historical Outline* (Philadelphia: 1897), 89–142.
7. Cora B. Marrett, "On the Evolution of Women's Medical Studies," *Bulletin of the History of Medicine* 53 (Fall 1979): 434–48.
8. See *Transactions of the Alumnae Association of the Woman's Medical College of Pennsylvania* (Philadelphia: 1875–1921); Regina Markell Morantz, "Bertha Van Hoosen," in *Notable American Women: The Modern Period,* ed. B. Sicherman and C. Hurd Green (Cambridge, MA: Harvard University Press, 1980), 706–7.
9. See Walsh, *"Doctors Wanted,"* 178–267; William Chafe, *The American Woman* (New York: Oxford University Press, 1972), 89–112; Barbara Harris, *Beyond Her Sphere: Women and the Professions in American History* (Westport, CT: Greenwood Press, 1978), 95–126.
10. Chafe, *The American Woman,* 90; Walsh, *"Doctors Wanted,"* 186.
11. Rosemary Stevens, *American Medicine and the Public Interest* (New Haven, CT: Yale University Press, 1971), 55–73; David Rosner and Gerald Markowitz, "Doctors in Crisis: Medical Education and Medical Reform During the Progressive Era, 1895–1915," *American Quarterly* 25 (March 1973): 83–107.
12. See E. Richard Brown, *Rockefeller Medicine Men: Medicine and Capitalism in America* (Berkeley: University of California Press, 1979); Eliot Friedson, *Profession of Medicine* (New York: Dodd, Mead, 1970); Megali Larson, *The Rise of Professionalism* (Berkeley: University of California Press, 1977); Burton J. Bledstein, *The Culture of Professionalism* (New York: W. W. Norton, 1978); Stevens, *American Medicine*; and Rosner and Markowitz, "Doctors in Crisis." It should be noted that these "revisionist" medical historians are taking part in a respectable and longstanding debate among American historians on the subject of how progressive and reformist was progressive reform. James R. Burrow has argued recently that the medical profession was in favor of social reform during the

progressive era, but I would contend that the issue is still very much open to contention. See James Burrow, *Organized Medicine in the Progressive Era* (Baltimore: Johns Hopkins University Press, 1977).

13. Stevens, *American Medicine,* 58–68, 69.

14. Editorial, *Journal of the American Medical Association* 35 (August 1900): 501, quoted in Rosner and Markowitz, "Doctors in Crisis," 98. Emphasis added.

15. Stevens, *American Medicine,* 68; also Robert P. Hudson, "Abraham Flexner in Perspective: American Medical Education, 1865–1910," *Bulletin of the History of Medicine* 56 (November–December 1972): 545–61.

16. These three schools were the Woman's Medical College of Pennsylvania, the Woman's Medical College of Baltimore, and the New York Medical College for Women, a homeopathic institution. For the Philadelphia college's financial problems, see Gulielma Fell Alsop, *A History of the Woman's Medical College* (Philadelphia: J. B. Lippincott, 1950). Black medical schools suffered the same fate.

17. For a good discussion of discrimination, see Walsh, *"Doctors Wanted,"* 178–267, and Gloria Melnick Moldow, "The Gilded Age, Promise and Disillusionment: Women Doctors and the Emergence of the Professional Middle Class, Washington, D.C., 1870–1900" (Ph. D. diss., University of Maryland, 1980), 88–130, 163–90.

18. See Regina Markell Morantz, "Science vs. Art: The Medical Thought of Mary Putnam Jacobi and Elizabeth Blackwell" (Paper delivered at the American Association of the History of Medicine Conference, Boston, Massachusetts, May 1980).

19. See Regina Markell Morantz, "Women Physicians, Co-education and the Struggle for Professional Standards in 19th-Century Medical Education" (Paper delivered at Berkshire Conference, Mount Holyoke College, South Hadley, MA, August 1978).

20. For Blackwell's arguments, see "The New York Infirmary and Medical College for Women," in *Transactions of the Alumnae Association of the Woman's Medical College of Pennsylvania, 1900,* 76–80. For Flexner, see Abraham Flexner, *Medical Education in the United States and Canada* (New York: The Carnegie Foundation, 1910), 296, 178–79.

21. Carol Lopate, *Women in Medicine* (Baltimore: Johns Hopkins University Press, 1968), 17.

22. Walker to Van Hoosen, February 6, 1940, Van Hoosen Papers, Medical College of Pennsylvania Archives. Hereinafter, papers from the Medical College of Pennsylvania Archives are cited as MCP.

23. See Charles Rosenberg, "The Therapeutic Revolution: Medicine, Meaning, and Social Change in Nineteenth-Century America," *Perspectives in Biology and Medicine* 20 (Summer 1977): 485–506.

24. This description of modern therapeutics relies on Edmund D. Pellegrino, M.D., "From the Rational to the Radical: The Sociocultural Impact of Modern Therapeutics" in *The Therapeutic Revolution: Essays in the Social History of American Medicine,* ed. Morris Vogel and Charles Rosenberg (Philadelphia: University of Pennsylvania Press, 1979); and George L. Engel, "The Need for a New Medical Model: A Challenge for Biomedicine," *Science* 196 (April 1977): 129–35.

25. Stevens, *American Medicine,* 77–79. Morris Vogel, "The Transformation of the American Hospital" in *Health Care in America,* ed. David Rosner and Susan Reverby (Philadelphia: Temple University Press, 1979), 105–16.

26. Elizabeth Gregg, "The Tuberculosis Nurse under Municipal Direction," *Public Health Nursing Quarterly* 5 (October 1913): 16. I am indebted to Dr. Barbara Bates for this citation.

27. Eliza Mosher, "The Human in Medicine, Surgery and Nursing," *Woman's Medical*

Journal 32 (May 1925): 117–19. See also Emily Dunning Barringer, *Bowery to Bellevue* (New York: W. W. Norton, 1950), 244, and Josephine Baker, *Fighting for Life* (New York: Macmillan, 1959), 248.

28. Harding to Van Hoosen, May 6, 1930, Van Hoosen Papers, MCP.

29. L. Powers, H. Wiesenfelder, and R. C. Parmelee, "Practice Patterns of Men and Women Physicians," *Journal of Medical Education* 44 (January–June 1969): 481–91.

30. Walsh, *"Doctors Wanted,"* 259.

31. See Adelaide Brown, M.D., *What Medicine Offered in 1888 and Now in 1938,* pamphlet reprinted from *Woman's City Club Magazine* (August 1938), Sophia Smith Collection; Hulda Thelander and Helen B. Weyrauch, "Women in Medicine," *Journal of the American Medical Woman's Association* 148 (February 1952): 531–34. For women's work with the Children's Bureau see Nancy P. Weiss, "Save the Children: A History of the Children's Bureau, 1903–1918" (Ph.D. diss., University of California, 1974) and the papers of Dr. Dorothy Reed Mendenhall, Sophia Smith Collection. Also Mabel Ulrich, "Men Are Queer That Way: Extracts From the Diary of an Apostate Woman Physician," *Scribner's Magazine* 93 (June 1933): 365–69.

32. See Josephine Baker, *Fighting for Life*; Alice Hamilton, *Exploring the Dangerous Trades* (Boston: Little, Brown, 1943); see also Ellen C. Potter Manuscripts, MCP; Gert Brieger, "Florence Sabin," *Notable American Women: The Modern Period,* 614–16.

33. Rosner and Markowitz, "Doctors in Crisis," 89.

34. Statistics on the numbers of women graduate students are taken from the *Records of the Commissioner of Education, 1894–95, 1910, 1915, 1918.* Statistics on women welfare workers, "physicians' and surgeons' attendants," and "keepers of charitable and penal institutions" are taken from U.S. Bureau of Census, *U.S. Census of Population* (Washington, D. C.: U.S. Government Printing Office, 1900, 1910, 1920).

35. Harris, *Beyond Her Sphere,* 101.

36. Henry P. May, *The End of American Innocence* (New York: Knopf, 1959); William L. O'Neill, *Divorce in the Progressive Era* (New Haven, CT: Yale University Press, 1967); James R. McGovern, "The American Woman's Pre-World War I Freedom in Manners and Morals," *Journal of American History* 55 (September 1968): 315–33; Regina Markell Morantz, "The Scientist as Sex Crusader: Alfred Kinsey and American Culture," *American Quarterly* 29 (Winter 1977): 563–89; Sheila M. Rothman, *Women's Proper Place* (New York: Basic Books, 1978); and John Burnham, "The Progressive Era Revolution in Attitudes Toward Sex," *Journal of American History* 59 (March 1973): 885–908.

37. Harris, *Beyond Her Sphere,* 134.

38. Joyce Antler, "Feminism as Life Process: The Life and Career of Lucy Sprague Mitchell," *Feminist Studies* 7 (Spring 1981): 134–57.

39. Ibid., 135; Frank Stricker, "Cookbooks and Law Books: The Hidden History of the Career Woman in 20th-Century America," *Journal of Social History* 10 (Fall 1976): 1–19.

40. Mabel Gardner, M.D., to Catherine Macfarlane, M.D., February 4, 1952. Macfarlane Manuscripts, MCP.

41. See in this regard Mabel Ulrich, "Men Are Queer That Way."

42. Lopate, *Women in Medicine,* 193–95; C. Nadelson and M. Notman, "The Woman Physician," *Journal of Medical Education* 47 (March 1972): 176–83.

43. Kristine Mann, M.D., "Medical Women's Handicap," *Harper's Weekly* 58 (February 1914): 32; Editorials, "Women in Medicine," *Journal of American Medical Women's Association* 1 (April 1946): 93–95.

This Promised Land:

Women Doctors One Hundred Years Later

RUTH J. ABRAM

It is for you to enter this Promised Land, this land of equal opportunity.
–Dr. Elizabeth Carpenter, 1919

HOW have women physicians advanced in the last century in this "land of equal opportunity"? Below, we compare the results of Dr. Rachel Bodley's 1881 survey of the graduates of the Woman's Medical College of Pennsylvania with the results of more recent surveys.

Are you now engaged in active medical practice?

I. Rate of Attrition

1881: 87% of Bodley's respondents "responded affirmatively."
1981: 92.5% of women physicians were in active practice.[H]

II. Type of Practice

1881: The majority of Bodley's respondents were involved in gynecology and obstetrics.
1981: Women physicians' specialities were internal medicine (16%), pediatrics (15%), general practice (9%). Obstetrics and gynecology accounted for only 6% of the work of all female practitioners.[E]

What is the predominating character of [your] medical practice?

III. Social Reception

1881: 96% of Bodley's respondents reported "cordial social recognition."

[What is] the social status of the woman physician in the

community in which she dwells?

1976: Responding to a 1976 Gallup poll, 58% of men and 49% of women said they preferred male physicians. 40% of both sexes had no preference.[H]

The work . . . accomplished by the woman practitioner as resident or visiting physician in hospital, asylum, charitable institution or as physician in college or school for girls is inspiriting.

IV. Institutional Practice

1881: 38% of Bodley's respondents were thus engaged.
1981: 35% of all female physicians were in hospital-based practice, either as residents (25%) or as full-time hospital staff (10%).[E]

[What is the] monetary value of the practice per year?

V. Income

1881: Bodley's respondents reported an average annual income of $2,907 (compare to average annual income of $244 in 1880).
1983: *Medica* magazine's 1983 survey reported an average annual income of $50,500 (compare to average annual per capital income of $9,510 in 1980).[M]

Are you a member of a county, state or other local medical society?

VI. Medical Societies

1881: 36% of Bodley's respondents "reply affirmatively."
1981: 33% of all female physicians are members of the A.M.A.

What influence has the study and practice of medicine had upon your domestic relations as wife and mother?

—Dr. Rachel Bodley

VII. Combining Career and Family

1881: 87% of Bodley's respondents "reply favorable."
1983: A survey of women physicians conducted by *Medica* magazine in 1983 found that 57% of all women physicians were married, 70% had children, 14% had been divorced.[M]

Reading between the lines of her survey, Dr. Rachel Bodley concluded, "These statistics emphasize cheerful contentment. [The woman physician] has found her calling in life. It is soul satisfying."

A century later, 60% of women physicians responding to a Harris poll said they would recommend the practice of medicine to others, as compared with 50% of the male physicians.

In 1984, over 21,000 women were enrolled in medical school, representing 32% of all enrollees. Dr. Marilyn Heins attributes this unprecedented increase to three major factors: enactment of federal antidiscrimination legislation, adoption of a resolution on equal opportunity by the Assembly of the Association of American Medical Colleges (November 1970), and changes in women's attitudes and aspirations engendered by the feminist movement.[H]

The Promised Land seems once again in view—once again.

NOTES

H: Heins, Marilyn, M.D., "Update: Women in Medicine." *Journal of the American Medical Women's Association,* March/April 1985.
E: Eiler, Mary Ann, Ph.D., "Physician Characteristics and Distribution in the United States," American Medical Association, 1983.
M: *Medica, Women Practicing Medicine,* Fall 1983, "1983 Medica Survey of Women Physicians."

APPENDIX

Index

Page numbers in *italics* refer to illustrations.

INDEX